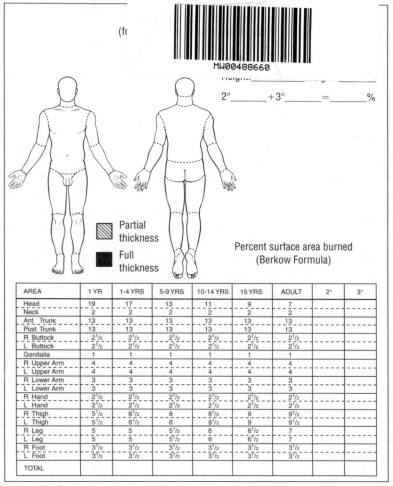

(f...

2° _____ +3° _____ = _____ %

Partial thickness

Full thickness

Percent surface area burned
(Berkow Formula)

AREA	1 YR	1-4 YRS	5-9 YRS	10-14 YRS	15 YRS	ADULT	2°	3°
Head	19	17	13	11	9	7		
Neck	2	2	2	2	2	2		
Ant Trunk	13	13	13	13	13	13		
Post Trunk	13	13	13	13	13	13		
R Buttock	2$^1/_2$	2$^1/_2$	2$^1/_2$	2$^1/_2$	2$^1/_2$	2$^1/_2$		
L Buttock	2$^1/_2$	2$^1/_2$	2$^1/_2$	2$^1/_2$	2$^1/_2$	2$^1/_2$		
Genitalia	1	1	1	1	1	1		
R Upper Arm	4	4	4	4	4	4		
L Upper Arm	4	4	4	4	4	4		
R Lower Arm	3	3	3	3	3	3		
L Lower Arm	3	3	3	3	3	3		
R Hand	2$^1/_2$	2$^1/_2$	2$^1/_2$	2$^1/_2$	2$^1/_2$	2$^1/_2$		
L Hand	2$^1/_2$	2$^1/_2$	2$^1/_2$	2$^1/_2$	2$^1/_2$	2$^1/_2$		
R Thigh	5$^1/_2$	6$^1/_2$	8	8$^1/_2$	9	9$^1/_2$		
L Thigh	5$^1/_2$	6$^1/_2$	8	8$^1/_2$	9	9$^1/_2$		
R Leg	5	5	5$^1/_2$	6	6$^1/_2$	7		
L Leg	5	5	5$^1/_2$	6	6$^1/_2$	7		
R Foot	3$^1/_2$	3$^1/_2$	3$^1/_2$	3$^1/_2$	3$^1/_2$	3$^1/_2$		
L Foot	3$^1/_2$	3$^1/_2$	3$^1/_2$	3$^1/_2$	3$^1/_2$	3$^1/_2$		
TOTAL								

Data from Berkow SG. A method of estimating the extensiveness of lesions (burns and scalds) based on surface area proportions. Arch Surg 8:138-148, 1924; and Lund CC, Browder NC. The estimation of areas of burns. Surg Gynecol Obstet 79:352-358, 1944.

AMERICAN BURN ASSOCIATION CRITERIA FOR INJURIES REQUIRING REFERRAL TO A BURN CENTER

- Partial-thickness burns of greater than 10% of the body surface area (BSA)
- Burns that involve the face, hands, feet, genitalia, perineum, or major joints
- Third-degree burns in any age group
- Electrical burns, including lightning injury
- Chemical burns
- Inhalation injury
- Burn injury in patients with preexisting medical disorders that could complicate management, prolong recovery, or affect mortality
- Any patient with burns and concomitant trauma (such as fractures), in whom the burn injury poses the greatest risk of morbidity or mortality. In such cases, if the trauma poses the greater immediate risk, the patient may be initially stabilized in a trauma center before being transferred to a burn unit. Physician judgment will be necessary and should be in concert with the regional medical control plan and triage protocols.
- Burned children in hospitals that do not have qualified personnel or equipment for the care of children
- Burn injury in patients who will require special social, emotional, or rehabilitation intervention

The Essential
Burn Unit Handbook

The Essential Burn Unit Handbook
SECOND EDITION

Jeffrey J. Roth, MD

Las Vegas Plastic Surgery
Las Vegas, Nevada

William B. Hughes, MD

Director, Temple University Hospital Burn Unit
Philadelphia, Pennsylvania

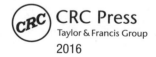

CRC Press
Taylor & Francis Group
2016

CRC Press
Taylor & Francis Group
6000 Broken Sound Parkway NW, Suite 300
Boca Raton, FL 33487-2742

© 2016 by Taylor & Francis Group, LLC
CRC Press is an imprint of Taylor & Francis Group, an Informa business

No claim to original U.S. Government works

Printed and bound in India by Replika Press Pvt. Ltd.

Printed on acid-free paper
Version Date: 20150811

International Standard Book Number-13: 978-1-4987-0571-4 (Pack - Book and Ebook)

Visit the Taylor & Francis Web site at
http://www.taylorandfrancis.com

and the CRC Press Web site at
http://www.crcpress.com

To my wife, *Dena,*
and my daughter, *Caroline,*
and to the memory of my mother,
Carol Ann Roth, RN

J.J.R.

. . .

To my wife, *Michelle,*
and my sons, *Liam* and *Kevin*

W.B.H.

EXECUTIVE EDITOR   Sue Hodgson
DEVELOPMENTAL EDITOR, MEDICAL   Megan Fennell
SENIOR PROJECT EDITING MANAGER   Carolyn Reich
MANAGING EDITOR   Suzanne Wakefield
EDITOR/PROJECT MANAGER   Glenn Floyd
PRODUCTIONISTS   Chris Lane, Debra Clark, Elaine Kitsis
GRAPHICS MANAGER   Brett Stone
DIRECTOR OF MEDICAL ILLUSTRATION   Brenda Bunch
PROOFREADER   Linda Maulin
INDEXER   Nancy Newman

Preface

The Philadelphia Burn Unit, located in Temple University Hospital, has dedicated its services to the care of injured patients since 1974. Inpatient admissions average 200 per year, with 2700 outpatient visits annually. The *Essential Burn Unit Handbook* is based on treatments that have evolved over a period of years and are at this time the standard of care at the burn center.

As residents serving in the Philadelphia Burn Unit, we were blessed with an outstanding nursing staff, established protocols that were tempered with experience, and attending surgeons who understood the plight of the house officer. They taught us well, and they gave us the necessary latitude to mature, gain confidence, and test our mettle.

Yet we felt there had to be a better way to obtain the essential knowledge base quickly. We tried various textbooks, but we could not find concise answers to urgent issues in any one source, and the information we did find was not portable to the ER, OR, burn unit, rehab unit, trauma bay, clinic, or ward. We have been in the situation in which you alone have to make decisions about the management of your patient, and where you must do the best you can with the tools available to you. It became clear to us that the oral tradition in which the chief resident imparts knowledge, experience, and pearls needed to be written down for the benefit of junior house officers, students, and everyone on the burn team.

This handbook represents our effort to fill a void and to communicate the common practices and workings of an active burn unit, with the rationales behind them and sample protocols to guide treatment. Our goal is to enhance the educational experience of the house officer rotating through the burn unit so that he or she can concentrate on care of the patient.

This second edition covers the spectrum of burn care, from initial assessment and treatment to long-term sequelae. We have added a chapter on the criteria for admissions to a burn unit and outpatient and follow-up care. The book includes a wealth of topics that surgical residents, emergency medicine residents, and critical care fellows will encounter. These include nutrition, antibiotics, wound care, and some of the unique pathologic conditions seen in this unique and often critically injured patient population. There is content on inhalation injury and electrical and chemical burns, as well as pediatric patient management. Health care personnel involved in the care of burn patients, including dietitians, occupational therapists, physical therapists, nurses, EMTs, respiratory therapists, and medical and nursing students, will benefit from reading this book. The handbook also includes sample orders and templates for patient presentation and organization of notes. The appendix includes a glossary for quick reference to the many acronyms and abbreviations used in this setting and a list of useful equations and ranges.

It is our hope that this book will help residents to provide better patient care and will shorten the learning curve. This concise, pocket-sized manual goes beyond the popular surgical house officer handbooks, presenting more of the day-to-day management modalities.

The treatment of burn patients is constantly evolving, and new techniques and modalities are being evaluated continually. Each patient represents a unique challenge, and therapy must be planned and tailored to the individual patient from the time of admission. Some protocols may vary from hospital to hospital—as in all of medicine, there may be more than one way to do things—but it is important to recognize that the principles remain the same.

Jeffrey J. Roth
William B. Hughes

Acknowledgments

We would like to acknowledge the contributions to this book of Dr. Frederick A. DeClement, Jr., Director of the Philadelphia Burn Unit, Emeritus, who has more than 30 years of experience in the care of burned patients. He has been our professor, mentor, and friend.

We would like to thank those who trained us, those who supported us during our training, and those who continue to support us daily as we attempt to apply what we have learned to our patients' care.

We would also like to thank the team at Quality Medical Publishing, particularly Karen Berger, Suzanne Wakefield, and Susan Trail, for helping to make the original book a reality. We would also like to thank the team at Taylor & Francis Group, CRC Press, particularly Sue Hodgson, Megan Fennell, Carolyn Reich, and Glenn Floyd, for helping to make the second edition a reality.

The first edition of *The Essential Burn Unit Handbook* has been used for more than 10 years by the residents in our programs and now varied programs. Thankfully, they continue to be enthusiastic about the book and say that it has made their job easier; they particularly cite the clear explanations. We have incorporated many of their suggestions into this second edition.

For such residents this book was written—for the ones called to a patient's bedside at 2 AM. If this book in some small way helps you, and in turn helps your patient, then we have accomplished what we set out to do, and our efforts have been worthwhile.

Please contact us with your questions, comments, and suggestions. We look forward to hearing from you.

Contents

1 ■ Introduction to the Burn Unit **1**

2 ■ Pathophysiology **5**

3 ■ Evaluation, Resuscitation, and Treatment **14**

4 ■ Admissions and Follow-up Care **48**

5 ■ Wound Care, Use of Antibiotics, and Control of Burn Wound Sepsis **54**

6 ■ Nutrition **68**

7 ■ Inhalation Injury **85**

8 ■ General (Nonburn) Inpatient Wound Care **103**

9 ■ Toxic Epidermal Necrolysis Syndrome and Stevens-Johnson Syndrome **128**

10 ■ Electrical Burns **138**

11 ■ Chemical Burns **144**

12 ■ Pediatric Burn Management **152**

Appendix **173**

Index **180**

The Essential
Burn Unit Handbook

1 Introduction to the Burn Unit

KEY POINTS

- More than 1 million burn injuries and more than 3000 deaths from burns occur each year in the United States.
- The rate of burn injuries has decreased.
- More than 60% of admissions are to burn centers.

A burn patient is a unique challenge for the clinician. Burns are common injuries and represent a significant medical, social, and economic problem. In the United States, an estimated 1.2 million burn injuries occur each year.[1-7] There are 3400 fire/burn/smoke inhalation deaths per year. This total includes 2550 deaths from residential fires, 300 from vehicle crash fires, and 550 from other sources (approximately 150 deaths from flame burns or smoke inhalation in nonresidential fires and 400 from contact with electricity, scalding liquids, and hot objects). Fire and burn deaths are combined in these statistics, because deaths from burns in fires cannot always be distinguished from deaths from toxic smoke or other nonburn causes.[4,8] In 2013 there was one civilian fire death every 2 hours and 42 minutes, and one civilian fire injury every 33 minutes. This represents a decrease in fatalities of 20.6% from 2002 to 2011.[4] Trend analysis indicates a decrease of 78% in civilian fire fatalities and a decrease of 68% in civilian fire injuries per capita from 1977 to 2012.[9]

1

There are 700,000 emergency room visits annually in the United States for burn injury. More than 80% of the U.S. population lives within 2 hours (by ground transport) of a verified burn center.[10] Most burn patients can safely be transported on the ground to a specialized burn center for their care. Some patients are too unstable to travel long distances; referring facilities can work with the burn center to stabilize and prepare these patients for a safe transfer.[11]

Approximately 40,000 inpatient acute hospitalizations are related to burn injury (Box 1-1). This includes 30,000 at hospital burn centers. More than 60% of the estimated U.S. acute hospitalizations related to burn injury were admitted to 127 burn centers. Such centers now average over 200 annual admissions for burn injury and skin disorders requiring similar treatment. The other 4500 U.S. acute care hospitals average less than three burn admissions per year.[12,13]

The economic impact is significant: a burn of 30% of total body area can cost $200,000 for initial hospitalization costs and physicians' fees. For extensive burns, additional significant costs are incurred, including costs for repeat admissions for reconstruction and rehabilita-

---

Box 1-1
Admissions to U.S. Burn Centers (ABA National Burn Repository 2014): Statistics for 2003 to 2012

Survival rate:	96.7%
Sex:	69% male, 31% female
Ethnicity:	59% white, 20% black, 14% Hispanic, 7% other
Admission cause:	43% fire/flame, 34% scald, 9% contact, 4% electrical, 3% chemical, 7% other
Place of occurrence:	73% home, 8% occupational, 5% street/highway, 5% recreational/sport, 9% other

Data from American Burn Association. Burn Incidence and Treatment in the United States: 2014 Fact Sheet; and American Burn Association. 2014 National Burn Repository Report of Data From 2004-2013. Chicago, The Association, 2014.

tion.[3,14] For severe burns treated without complications, the average cost significantly tops the million dollar mark at $1,617,345. With complications, a patient with a severe burn can cost more than $10 million to treat successfully.[6,7] These injuries cost the United States more than $18 billion per year.[15]

Although the numbers are impressive, the most important issue is the patient. A burn center is an ideal place for treating patients with thermal, chemical, electrical, and other significant cutaneous injuries. Staff members are well trained and comfortable treating patients with massive cutaneous injuries and the concomitant systemic effects. The physical plant is also conducive to the treatment and comfort of these patients. Together, all of these benefits decrease mortality and morbidity. Some burn centers have different protocols and achieve excellent results.

This book provides insight into treatments that have tended to work in our burn center and the rationale for their use. The world of burn surgery and critical care is always changing; this is a challenge and also part of the excitement, because a new technology or technique may make a large difference. Caring for this unique population is a very powerful experience.

REFERENCES

1. Baker SP, O'Neill B, Ginsberg NJ, et al. Fire, burns, and lightning. In Baker SP, O'Neill B, Ginsberg NJ, et al, eds. The Injury Fact Book, ed 2. New York: Oxford University Press, 1992.
2. National Center for Health Statistics. National Health Interview Survey (1991-1993).
3. American Burn Association. Burn Incidence and Treatment in the US: 2015 Fact Sheet. Chicago: The Association, 2015.
4. Karter MJ Jr. Fire Loss in the United States During 2013. Quincy, MA: National Fire Protection Association, Fire Analysis and Research Division, 2014.
5. National Center for Health Statistics. Annual Vital and Health Statistics Reports (to 1994). Atlanta, GA: Centers for Disease Control and Prevention, 1995.

6. The Burn Foundation. Burn Incidence and Treatment in the United States. Upland, PA: The Burn Foundation. Available at *http://www.burnfoundation. org/programs/resource.cfm?c=2&a=6.*

7. Centers for Disease Control and Prevention. National Hospital Ambulatory Medical Care Survey, and National Medical Expenditure Survey. Atlanta, GA: CDC, 2010.

8. National Safety Council. Injury Facts, 2014 edition. Itasca, IL: Research and Safety Management Solutions Group, 2014.

9. US Department of Homeland Security. Federal Emergency Management Agency. US Fire Administration. Fiscal Years 2012 and 2013: Report to Congress, Washington, DC, Oct 2014.

10. Klein MB, Kramer CB, Nelson J, et al. Geographic access to burn centers. JAMA 302:1774-1781, 2009.

11. Ortiz-Pujols SM, Thompson K, Sheldon GF, et al. Burn care: are there sufficient providers and facilities? Health Policy Research Institute. Bull Am Coll Surg 96:33-37, 2011.

12. Agency for Healthcare Research and Quality. National Inpatient Sample (HCUP-NIS: 2010 data).

13. Centers for Disease Control and Prevention. National Hospital Discharge Survey (2010 data). Atlanta, GA: CDC, 2011.

14. US Department of Labor. Bureau of Labor Statistics. Burn Statistics for 2013. Washington, DC: The Bureau, 2014.

15. President of the United States of America. Proclamation of National Burn Awareness Week, 2001. The White House, Office of the Press Secretary, Washington, DC, Feb 7, 2001.

2 Pathophysiology

ANATOMY

The average adult skin surface area is 1.5 to 2.0 square meters; in a newborn, the skin surface area is 0.2 to 0.3 square meters. The epidermis and dermis together range in thickness from 1 to 2 mm. The epidermis can be 0.05 mm thick, as in the eyelid, to 1 mm thick, as in the soles of the feet. Skin is generally thicker in males than in females. It peaks in thickness at 30 to 40 years of age and then thins. The skin is derived from ectoderm and mesoderm. It has many important functions, such as protection, fluid/electrolyte homeostasis, and thermoregulation, as well as immunologic, sensory, and metabolic roles (e.g., vitamin D synthesis).

BURN CLASSIFICATION

Burns are classified into three degrees (Fig. 2-1).

- *First-degree burns* are limited to the epidermis and result in edema formation and pain.
- *Second-degree burns* are either superficial or deep. Superficial burn wounds involve the epidermis and outer layer of the dermis. Generally, most of the dermal appendages (hair and glands) are spared. These wounds are painful, blisters occur, and the burns blanch with pressure. They are edematous and slippery to the touch because of proteinaceous exudate.[1] Deep second-degree burns involve most of the dermal appendages. Hairs fall out with a gentle pull, the wounds are white, edematous, blistered, and usually painless. Patients with deep second-degree burns may have a compromised blood supply to the dermis. They may sustain additional damage as a result of ischemia, free radical damage, and systemic alterations in the cytokine milieu of burn patients, leading to protein denaturation and necrosis. This may convert a second-degree burn to a third-degree burn.[2]
- *Third-degree burns* have disruption of all epithelial and dermal elements. They are depressed and nonedematous because of the lack of vascularization. The wounds have a leathery touch and can appear white, brown, or black. They are typically anesthetic. No spontaneous epithelialization occurs.[3,4]

Fig. 2-1   The various depths of burn injury.

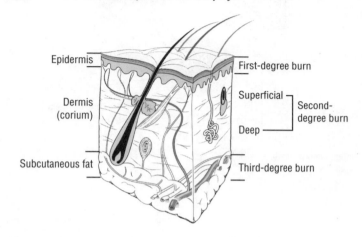

Epidermis

First-degree burn

Superficial ⎤
              ⎥ Second-
              ⎥ degree burn
Deep ─────────⎦

Dermis
(corium)

Subcutaneous fat

Third-degree burn

ZONES OF BURN INJURY

The effects of heat are temporal and quantitative. At temperatures of
40° to 44° C (104° to 111.2° F), enzymes malfunction, proteins denature, and cellular pumps fail. Above 44° C (111.2° F), the damage
occurs faster than the cell's repair mechanism can function. Damage
will continue even after the heat source is withdrawn, until the cooling process returns the skin to the normal range.

As proteins denature, cell necrosis progresses, and proteins alter
and coagulate. This occurs in the *zone of coagulation*, which is the first
of three zones used to describe the burn wound (Fig. 2-2). In this
zone, cell death is complete. It is usually the area nearest the heat
source, and this area forms the eschar of the burn wound.

Fig. 2-2   Zones of injury.

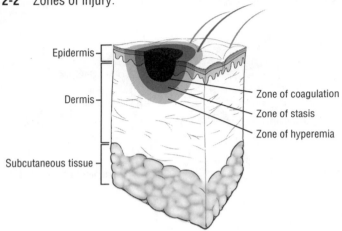

Superficial second-degree burn

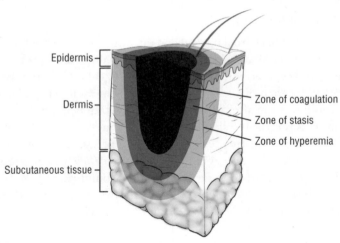

Deep second-degree burn

Below this is the *zone of stasis*. The cells are still viable, but circulation is impaired. As circulation is further compromised, ischemia results. Progressive vasoconstriction and thrombosis are seen; usually, this correlates with the severity of the primary injury.[5] These microvascular changes may lead to increased damage. The entire zone can become necrotic and turn into eschar if it does not heal.

The third zone is the *zone of hyperemia*. This area has minimal cellular injury but has predominant vasodilation, which increases blood flow. These cells usually recover.

PHYSIOLOGIC RESPONSE TO BURN INJURY

Burn edema and inflammation are caused by a variety of factors (Fig. 2-3). Generalized edema is usually seen in patients with burns greater than 30% total burned surface area (TBSA). The heat can directly damage vessels and increase permeability. Increased capillary permeability to protein is one of these changes. Equally important changes include the presence of an initial profound negative interstitial pressure "sucking" fluid into the tissues and a marked increase in interstitial space compliance. A host of mediators, especially oxidants, have been reported to cause these physical changes.[6] Heat alters proteins, which activates complement, which leads to histamine release and subsequent increased vessel permeability, causing thrombosis and activation of the coagulation systems. This leads to the release of serotonin (vasoconstriction) and bradykinin (increased permeability). Membrane phospholipids are altered or destroyed, which initiates the arachidonic acid cascade, leading to the release of leukotrienes (increase in permeability and neutrophil recruitment), thromboxane A_2 (vasoconstriction), prostacyclin (a vasodilator), and prostaglandins (increased dilation and constriction).

These mediators and hypoproteinemia may also increase interstitial edema throughout the body. Microvascular injury can interfere with the function of various organ systems.[5] Multiple organ system

Fig. 2-3   Physiologic response to burn. (*5-HPETE,* 5-hydroperoxyeico-satetraenoic acid; C_{3a}, complement component 3_a; C_{5a}, complement component 5_a; *LTA$_4$*, leukotriene A$_4$; *LTC$_4$*, leukotriene C$_4$; *LTD$_4$*, leukotriene D$_4$; *LTE$_4$*, leukotriene E$_4$; *PGD$_2$*, prostaglandin D$_2$; *PGE$_2$*, prostaglandin E$_2$; *PGF$_2$*, prostaglandin F$_2$; *PGG$_2$*, prostaglandin G$_2$; *PGH$_2$*, prostaglandin H$_2$; *PGI$_2$*, prostaglandin I$_2$.)

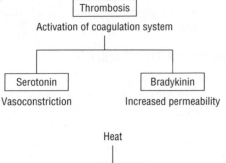

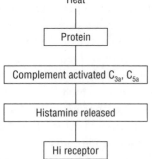

Intracellular gaps from actin-myosin contraction; protein leaks through gaps; ↑ tissue colloid oncotic pressure leads to fluid shift and edema formation in connective tissue and mucosa.

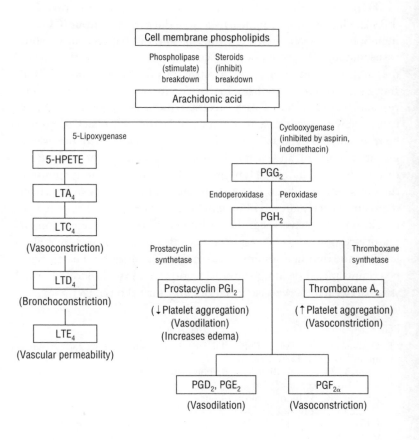

dysfunction can also occur from neutrophils sequestered in the lungs, liver, and other organs.[7-10]

Hypermetabolism is seen with a burn injury of greater than 20% TBSA. This response can nearly double the cardiac output (CO) and metabolic rate over the next 24 to 48 hours in patients successfully resuscitated. Hypermetabolism seems to peak at twice the normal metabolic rate in patients with burns of greater than 60% TBSA. Increased protein catabolism, increased gluconeogenesis, and insulin resistance are associated with this hypermetabolic response. The response may be secondary to a variety of factors. Feedback loops may be reset and the hypothalamus stimulated. This results in increases in glucagon, cortisol, and catecholamines. An increase in body temperature is also stimulated.[11] Hypermetabolism can occur in response to the evaporation of heat. In addition, the gut microbiota and environment are severely altered in patients with major burns. Abnormal gut conditions may have a significant influence on the systemic inflammatory response.[12] The response may also be influenced by a challenge to the immune system, because the gastrointestinal barrier may be compromised (leading to translocation), and the lack of a normal skin barrier may serve as a portal of entry for bacteria.[13-15]

REFERENCES

1. Widgerow AD, King K, Tocco-Tussardi I, et al. The burn wound exudate—an under-utilized resource. Burns 41:11-17, 2015.
2. Singh V, Devgan L, Bhat S, et al. The pathogenesis of burn wound conversion. Ann Plast Surg 59:109-115, 2007.
3. Kramer GC. Pathophysiology of burn shock and burn edema. In Herndon DN, ed. Total Burn Care, ed 4. Philadelphia: WB Saunders, 2012.
4. Jeffers L, Basu CB, eds. Plastic and Reconstructive Surgery: Essentials for Students, ed 8. Arlington Heights, IL: Plastic Surgery Educational Foundation, 2012.
5. Aggarwal SJ, Diller KR, Blake GK, et al. Burn-induced alterations in vasoactive function of the peripheral cutaneous microcirculation. J Burn Care Rehabil 15:1-12, 1994.

6. Demling RH. The burn edema process: current concepts. J Burn Care Rehabil 26:207-227, 2005.

7. Demling RH, LaLonde C, Liu Y, et al. The lung inflammatory response from thermal injury: relationship between physiological and histological changes. Surgery 106:52-59, 1989.

8. Evers LH, Bhavsar D, Mailänder P. The biology of burn injury. Exp Dermatol 19:777-783, 2010.

9. Lord JM, Midwinter MJ, Chen YF, et al. The systemic immune response to trauma: an overview of pathophysiology and treatment. Lancet 384:1455-1465, 2014.

10. Enkhbaatar P, Traber DL. Pathophysiology of acute lung injury in combined burn and smoke inhalation injury. Clin Sci (Lond) 107:137-143, 2004.

11. Youn YK, LaLonde C, Demling R. The role of mediators in the response to thermal injury. World J Surg 16:30-36, 1992.

12. Shimizu K, Ogura H, Asahara T, et al. Gut microbiota and environment in patients with major burns – a preliminary report. Burns 41:e28-e33, 2015.

13. Dietch EA. Multiple organ failure. Adv Surg 26:233-234, 1993.

14. Mozingo DW, McManus AT, Kim SH, et al. Incidence of bacteremia after burn wound manipulation in the early postburn period. J Trauma 42:1006-1010; discussion 1010-1011, 1997.

15. Bang RL, Sharma PN, Sanyal SC, et al. Burn septicaemia in Kuwait: associated demographic and clinical factors. Med Princ Pract 13:136-141, 2004.

3 Evaluation, Resuscitation, and Treatment

KEY POINTS

- Burn patients should be treated as trauma patients.
- An AMPLE history needs to be taken.
- Fluid resuscitation should be started.
- Patients are evaluated for escharotomy.
- Admission orders are placed.

INITIAL EVALUATION

A burn patient is by definition a trauma patient. One of the main objectives of the burn unit rotation for residents is to become familiar with this type of trauma, the pathophysiology, treatment modalities, and prognosis.

Residents should "ignore the burn" in the initial survey. With experience, they will not be intimidated by the burn, but will view the patient as any trauma patient. They should follow the steps necessary to treat any trauma patient and to address the issues in the proper sequence. The associated trauma may more quickly cause the patient's demise than the burn injury. Burn treatment starts as the ABCs of trauma are performed. This principle should prevail throughout the treatment course.[1]

INITIAL RESUSCITATION
History-Taking

The first step in the diagnosis and treatment of a burn patient is to obtain a detailed history of *a*llergies, *m*edications, *p*ast illnesses, *l*ast meal, and *e*vents preceding injury (AMPLE). This is extremely important. Helpful information may be obtained from the patient, witnesses, emergency personnel, and/or the fire marshal. Usually the first person to interview the patient has the best chance to document what actually happened to the patient.

The history should include the usual information, with attention to the mechanism of injury (e.g., the patient was involved in a motor vehicle accident or an explosion, or was trapped in a confined space) and the method of escape from the fire (e.g., the patient jumped from a second-story window). This will help to direct the search for concomitant injuries. The agent of the burn injury is also significant (e.g., a chemical, hydrofluoric acid, phosphorus, or butane).

The patient's past medical history, including allergies and medications, and surgical history are very important. Drug, alcohol, and smoking history should be noted. Documentation of these data is an essential part of history-taking. If the patient is able to communicate, the physician should ask the patient's height and weight. Most patients at least know this information, which is helpful for calculating the body surface area, the subsequent fluid rate, nutritional support, and drug dosages.

Many burns occur from attempted suicide, assault, and accidents that involve products or people. Some form of legal action will follow in more than 50% of these cases. This is another reason a detailed, legible history is important. The historian's name should be documented.[2]

Primary Survey

The burn itself should take a secondary role in the initial (primary) survey. Remember your A-B-C-D-Es.

AIRWAY   Is the airway patent? The airway is not compromised if the patient is talking normally. A hoarse voice or audible breathing (for example, stridor) is suspicious. Endotracheal intubation is the most definitive way to secure the airway. C-spine precautions are essential.

BREATHING   Is the patient moving air? Pneumothorax (tension or open), large hemothorax, and flail chest compromise breathing and should be treated with endotracheal intubation, mechanical ventilation, and/or tube thoracostomy as needed.

CIRCULATION   Does the patient have a blood pressure, and is it adequate to meet the patient's metabolic needs? Is the patient bleeding?

DISABILITY   Does the patient have any gross deformities (e.g., broken bones, neurologic deficits)? Penetrating injuries (both front and back) are noted. A neurologic examination is performed.

EXPOSURE   The patient is disrobed and examined, including the rectum. A Foley catheter is placed for accurate measurement of input and output. An NGT is placed for stomach decompression, ulcer prophylaxis, and enteral feedings.

Secondary Survey

AIRWAY   Is the face involved as a result of flame injury? Are blackened or charred areas present around the airway? Is carbonaceous sputum noted? Is soot present in the oropharynx? Is the patient able to clear his or her secretions? The physician should listen over the sternal notch.

BREATHING   Is the patient moving a sufficient amount of air? Is the patient hoarse? Is stridor present? Bronchoscopy is considered to document airway damage and swelling secondary to heat or toxins. In any inhalation injury or significant burn injury, intubation is a consideration. Patients with large burns may be talking on presentation, but this can change rapidly. This is especially important in light of the massive fluid resuscitation necessary, which may lead to edema at the oropharynx, causing upper airway obstruction. Intubation will protect the airway against delayed compromise resulting from injury that may not have been appreciated at the time of the initial examination. An escharotomy should be considered if the burns on the chest are full thickness and involve an entire anterior chest quadrant, or if the patient is not moving adequate volumes of air. If the wounds are partial-thickness burns, a chemical escharotomy with a proteolytic agent, such as Santyl, may be needed.

CIRCULATION   Pressure and signs of perfusion are monitored (warm knee caps, warm toes, and adequate urine output). IV access is secured with suturing for resuscitation; tape should not be used. Large-gauge peripheral lines are best used early in the resuscitation. Central access is needed for hemodynamic monitoring, drawing blood, and aggressive fluid resuscitation. The central access initially may be placed through the burn. This access should be sutured in four places to ensure stability. Maintenance of secure venous access is critical. In our protocol, the access will be changed in 3 days to decrease the potential for line sepsis and thrombus formation.

Burn edema accelerates with fluid resuscitation, making veins difficult to visualize, palpate, and cannulate. All rings, chains, and other items are removed, because they may constrict the patient when edema is present.

Edema will resolve when the microvascular system and the cell membranes recover from the thermal insult and resorption of the fluid from the extravascular space begins. This diuretic or mobilization phase usually occurs on the fourth to sixth day, but may extend for longer periods.

The physician should search for areas of hemorrhage and penetrating injuries and logroll the patient to inspect, palpate, and auscultate the back and spine. The patient's neck needs to be protected.

The patient is always rolled toward the first examiner, allowing the second examiner (on the other side) to examine the patient. The patient is then rolled toward the second examiner, allowing the first examiner to examine the patient. A CT scan may be necessary for evaluation.

DISABILITY   Potential traumatic injuries need to be addressed. This is especially important if the mechanism of injury was significant (e.g., auto accident, explosion, or traumatic escape). The patient is log-rolled and examined from head to toe. Palpation includes areas over bones. All areas are examined, including between the buttocks and the perineal area. Adequate lighting will facilitate the examination.

EXPOSURE   In the body diagram, the areas of burn are noted (Figs. 3-1 and 3-2). The burn is drawn, with the depth noted. The physician determines whether the burn extends across a joint or is circumferential. If the burn is a circumferential third-degree burn, an escharotomy may be necessary. The total burned surface area (TBSA) is estimated using Berkow's percentages chart (Fig. 3-3). As indicated on Fig. 3-3, partial-thickness burns get shaded with diagonal lines, and full-thickness burns get completely filled in. Now one can accurately add up the partial- and full-thickness burns to get the TBSA, and then make the necessary calculations.

Another convenient way of estimating the percentage of burn is to use the palmar surface of the patient's hand. The palmar surface (including the digits) can be estimated to be 1% (actually, it is 0.85%) of the body surface. The palmar surface of the hand minus the palmar area of the digits can be considered to be 0.5% of the body surface area (BSA).[3] In calculating the TBSA, first-degree burns are not included. The estimated percentage of burn is recorded in the appropriate space. This estimate may change after soot and dirt are removed in the tub room. Some areas of pigmented collapsed bullae of partial-thickness injury later may be debrided with dressing changes.

Fig. 3-1   Rule of nines: body diagram for estimating total burned surface area (%TBSA) in adults. (Numbers are for anterior only and posterior only.)

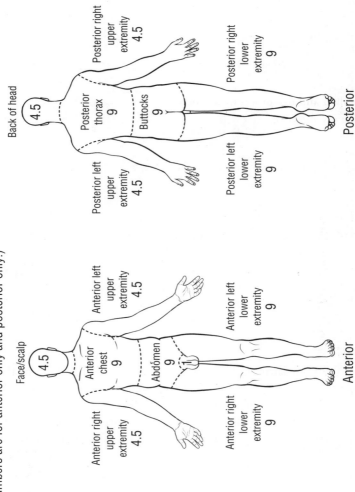

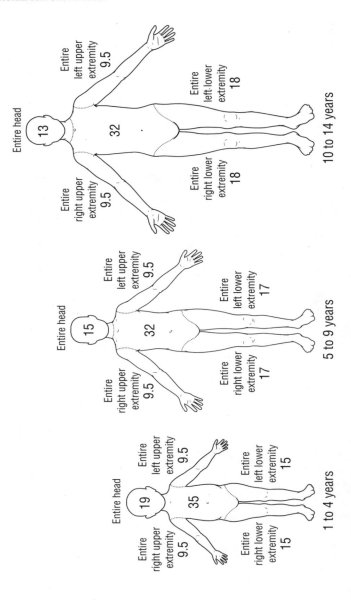

Fig. 3-2 Rule of nines, modified for pediatric patients: body diagram for estimating total burned surface area (%TBSA) in children. (Numbers include anterior and posterior.)

Fig. 3-3 Diagram and chart for estimating total burned surface area.
(Data from Berkow SG. A method of estimating the extensiveness of lesions [burns and scalds] based on surface area proportions. Arch Surg 8:138-148, 1924; and Lund CC, Browder NC. The estimation of areas of burns. Surg Gynecol Obstet 79:352-358, 1944.)

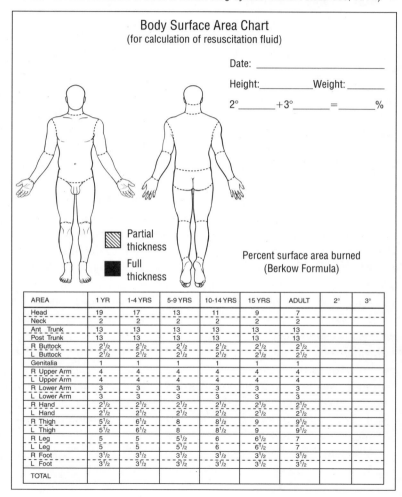

Body Surface Area Chart
(for calculation of resuscitation fluid)

Date: _____

Height:_____Weight: _____

$2°$_____$+3°$_____$=$_____%

Partial thickness

Full thickness

Percent surface area burned
(Berkow Formula)

AREA	1 YR	1-4 YRS	5-9 YRS	10-14 YRS	15 YRS	ADULT	2°	3°
Head	19	17	13	11	9	7		
Neck	2	2	2	2	2	2		
Ant. Trunk	13	13	13	13	13	13		
Post Trunk	13	13	13	13	13	13		
R Buttock	2½	2½	2½	2½	2½	2½		
L Buttock	2½	2½	2½	2½	2½	2½		
Genitalia	1	1	1	1	1	1		
R Upper Arm	4	4	4	4	4	4		
L Upper Arm	4	4	4	4	4	4		
R Lower Arm	3	3	3	3	3	3		
L Lower Arm	3	3	3	3	3	3		
R Hand	2½	2½	2½	2½	2½	2½		
L Hand	2½	2½	2½	2½	2½	2½		
R Thigh	5½	6½	8	8½	9	9½		
L Thigh	5½	6½	8	8½	9	9½		
R Leg	5	5	5½	6	6½	7		
L Leg	5	5	5½	6	6½	7		
R Foot	3½	3½	3½	3½	3½	3½		
L Foot	3½	3½	3½	3½	3½	3½		
TOTAL								

RESUSCITATION   The secondary survey includes resuscitation. We use the Parkland formula as a starting point for fluid resuscitation. The initial 24-hour fluid replacement with lactated Ringer's solution is calculated as follows:

$$4 \text{ ml} \times \text{Body weight in kilograms} \times$$
$$\% \text{ of Total burned surface area (\%TBSA) of the burn injury}$$
$$(\text{e.g., } 4 \text{ ml} \times 70 \text{ kg} \times 60\% \text{ burn} = 16{,}800 \text{ ml})$$

This can be done quickly using the *rule of nines* (see Fig. 3-1): The head, each upper extremity, the anterior chest, the posterior thorax, the abdomen, and the buttocks each equal approximately 9% of the TBSA in an adult. Each lower extremity is 18% of the TBSA. These percentages shift for pediatric patients (see Fig. 3-2). The more accurate and preferred way to estimate TBSA is to use the Berkow/Lund chart (see Fig. 3-3) for drawing the TBSA and calculating resuscitation fluids. Fluid resuscitation is calculated beginning from the time of injury, not when the patient arrives in the emergency department. The first half of this volume is to be administered within 8 hours of the burn (even if transfer of the patient to the medical center is delayed). The second half of the volume is given over the next 16 hours. A too-rapid decrease in the fluid resuscitation may result in hypotension and/or a decrease in the urinary output. Therefore we decrease the fluid volume by 50 to 100 ml/hr until the calculated dose is achieved. The calculations are a guide. Physicians should tailor the volume replacement to the patient. We use urine output as an indicator of the adequacy of fluid resuscitation. Acceptable urine output is usually 0.5 ml/kg/hr (usually 30 ml).[4] Personnel need to be mindful of the volume of fluid given in the trauma bay. Fluids given too quickly can lead to bowel edema and secondary abdominal compartment syndrome.[5-7]

After the first 24 hours, the maintenance fluid is ½ NS. The rate is calculated for 24 hours by using the guideline in Table 3-1.

Table 3-1 Method for Calculating Maintenance Fluid

First 10 kg	100 ml/kg
Second 10 kg	50 ml/kg
Every kilogram above 20 kg	20 ml/kg

For example, the rate for a 70 kg patient is calculated as follows:

$$[100 \times 10 \text{ (for the first 10 kg)}] + [50 \times 10 \text{ (for the second 10 kg)}] +$$
$$[20 \times 50 \text{ (for the 50 kilograms not yet covered)}]:$$
$$1000 \text{ ml} + 500 \text{ ml} + 1000 \text{ ml} = 2500 \text{ ml}/24 \text{ hr.}$$

The rate of maintenance fluids is 104 ml/hr. This is an estimate. The rate can be rounded up to a more manageable number (e.g., 105 ml/hr).

During the fourth 8-hour period after a burn, salt-poor albumin (SPA) is infused using the formula $0.1 \times \text{kilograms} \times \%\text{TBSA}$. The SPA is infused over 4 to 6 hours. This is given to increase oncotic pressure.[8]

Some burn units will administer free water in addition to the maintenance fluids for patients with more than 25% TBSA. Our unit will be mindful of the evaporative losses until the wound is covered. We typically add free water if the patient becomes hypernatremic. The calculation for water evaporation is:

$$\%\text{TBSA} + [25 \times \text{BSA in m}^2] = \text{Number of milliliters}$$
$$\text{of evaporative water loss/hr}$$

Remember that BSA should not be confused with TBSA. BSA is calculated as follows:

$$[87 (H + W) - 2600] \div 10{,}000 = \text{Surface in m}^2$$

where H = Height in cm; W = weight in kg. This amount is replaced as free water. Evaluation of serum Na will give an indication of adequate replacement. The optimal level of Na to be maintained is 135 to 137 mg/dl. As the slope of the curve of Na levels changes, trends can be determined and corrected before increased losses are present.

ASSESSMENT OF OTHER PARAMETERS

Trauma laboratory values, carboxyhemoglobin and arterial blood gas levels, a chest x-ray (CXR) evaluation, and ECG are obtained.

The patient is wrapped with warm blankets to prevent hypothermia. Covering the head will conserve significant amounts of heat. Hypothermia is secondary to the patient's skin loss. This regulatory barrier is now damaged, and the patient will lose heat by convection, conduction, radiation, and evaporation. This may occur subtly in a wet, undressed, hypotensive patient, despite routine monitoring. Dressings are placed to minimize heat and water losses and to keep antibacterial creams in contact with the burn injury.

WHAT'S NEXT

The patient will then undergo debridement in the burn center. This should take place in a room with warm ambient temperature (at least 28° C [82° F]). Escharotomy may be performed at this time if indicated, with electrocautery equipment; the patient is sedated intravenously. Escharotomy is performed on the medial and lateral surfaces of the extremities (Figs. 3-4 through 3-12), on the anterior axillary line, and subcostally on the chest (see Fig. 3-4). The incision is made down to the fat layer. In patients with little subcutaneous tissue, great care must be exercised to prevent inadvertent fasciotomy.

Large vessels injured during this process should be ligated with 4-0 ties. However, if the escharotomy is carefully performed, there should be little bleeding from the incised margins. Paradoxically, a pitfall of escharotomy is not making the incision deep enough. If dermal strands extend across the incision, the expansion of the tissue will be hampered.[9]

Text continued on p. 34.

Fig. 3-4 Escharotomy sites (whole body view).

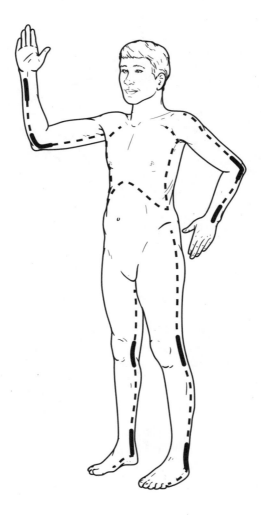

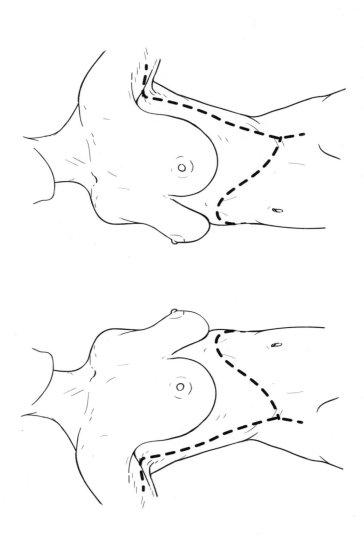

Fig. 3-5 Left and right trunk. *Dashed lines* indicate escharotomy incisions.

Fig. 3-6 Left and right hands. *Dashed lines* indicate escharotomy incisions.

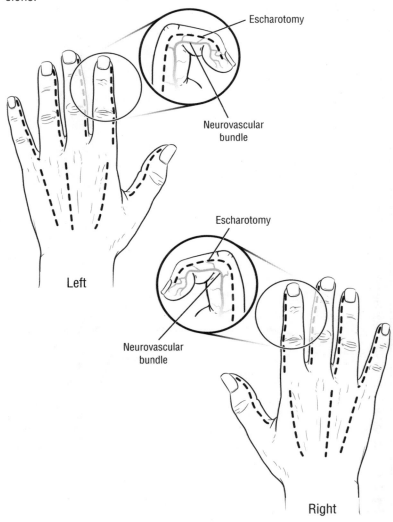

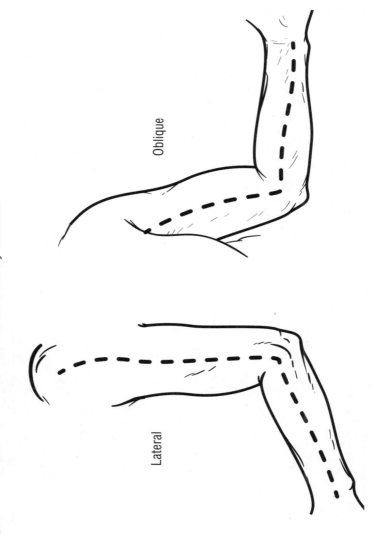

Fig. 3-7 Left elbow. *Dashed lines* indicate escharotomy incisions.

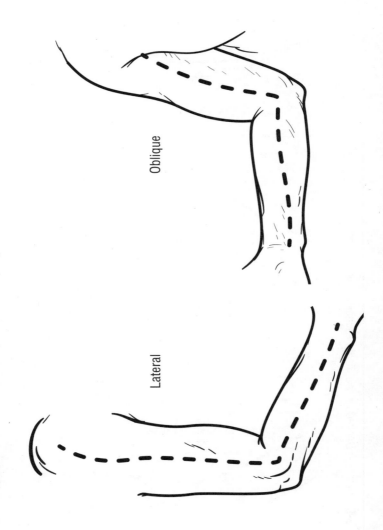

Fig. 3-8 Right elbow. *Dashed lines* indicate escharotomy incisions.

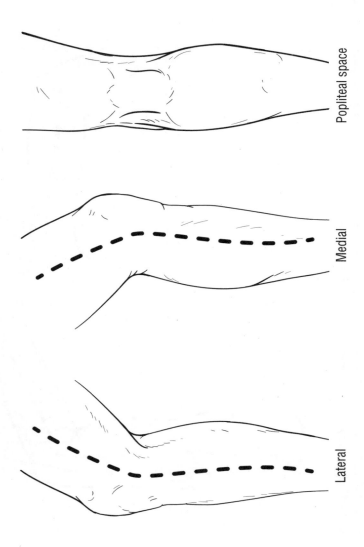

Fig. 3-9 Left leg. *Dashed lines* indicate escharotomy incisions.

Popliteal space

Medial

Lateral

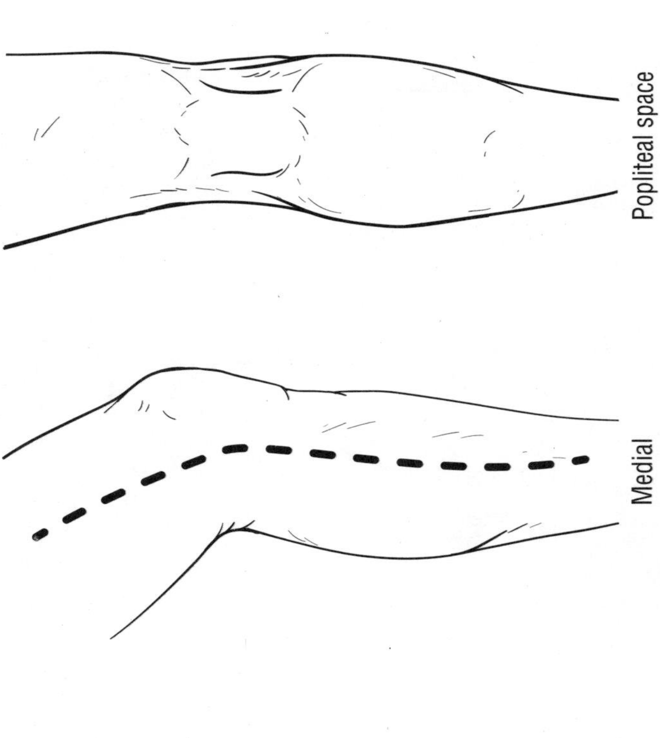

Fig. 3-10 Right leg. *Dashed lines* indicate escharotomy incisions.

Popliteal space

Medial

Lateral

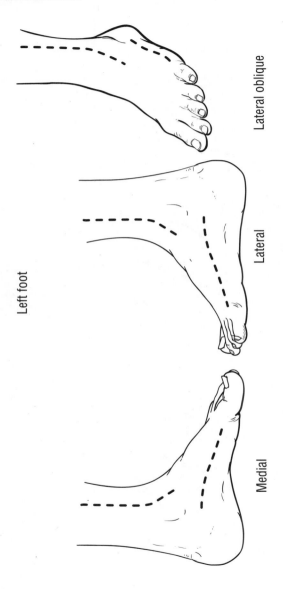

Fig. 3-11 Left foot. *Dashed lines* indicate escharotomy incisions.

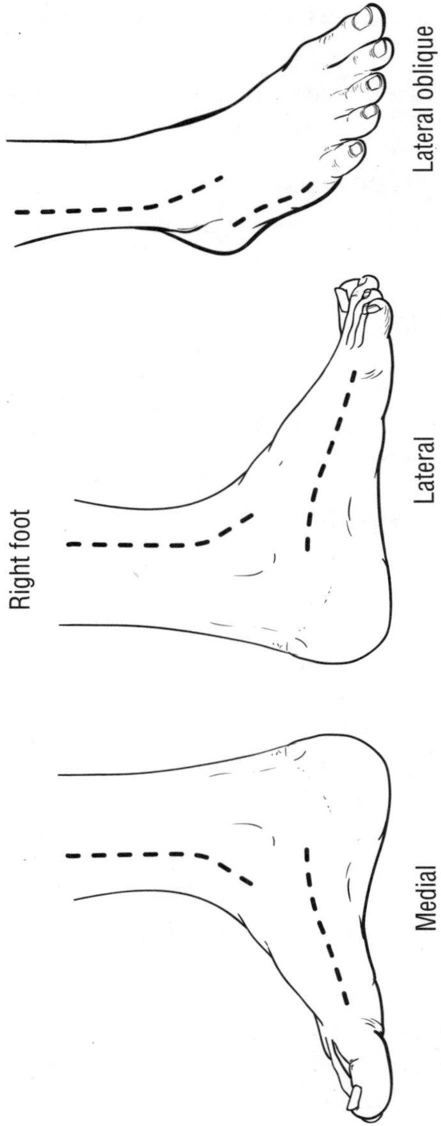

Fig. 3-12   Right foot. *Dashed lines* indicate escharotomy incisions.

Right foot

Lateral oblique

Lateral

Medial

ADMITTING A PATIENT TO THE BURN UNIT

The continuation of resuscitation, close monitoring, critical care, and wound care are best managed in a dedicated unit by personnel trained in the care of this unique patient population.[10-12]

Sample Admission Orders

(Do not write comments—shown here in italics—on the order sheet.)

ADMISSION

To burn unit

DX

s/p trauma, 50% TBSA burn secondary to falling asleep while smoking in bed.

HEIGHT AND WEIGHT

CONDITION

Critical

VITAL SIGNS

Per routine. [Continuous monitoring of vitals. Record qh; call HO if temp >39° C (102.5° F), P <60 or >100, BP <100 systolic or >160 systolic, pulse ox <90. Measure strict I&O qh; notify HO if <0.5 ml/kg/hr *(usually 30 ml/hr)*]. Monitor CVP; record qh.

ALLERGIES

(Document allergies and monitor drug interactions.)

ACTIVITY

Bed rest. Head of bed at 20 degrees *(to minimize cerebral and tracheal edema)*. No pillow for head and neck burns *(to minimize contractures and damage to ears)*.

NURSING

Per routine. Wound care as per unit protocol. *(See Chapter 5 for examples of such a protocol.)*

DIET

NPO if burn is >30%. Enteral feedings with TraumaCal or a similar formula. *(Target feedings of 25 kcal/kg/day times 2.0 [stress factor].)*

Tube feedings:

½ strength @ 25 ml/hr × 4 hr, then

¾ strength @ 25 ml/hr × 4 hr, then

Full strength @ 25 ml/hr × 4 hr, then

Increase 15 ml/q4h to goal.

Check residuals q4h; hold if >150 ml.

IV FLUIDS

Per Parkland formula. *(Give through a large-bore catheter sutured in place.)*

$$4 \text{ ml LR} \times \text{kg} \times \%\text{TBSA}$$

Give half in the first 8-hr period.

Give half in the next 16-hr period.

(Maintain urine output at 0.5-1.0 ml/kg/hr.)

If an inhalation injury is present in adults, the alteration may need to be 5 × kilograms × %TBSA. In an elderly patient or in children, the Parkland formula may need to be altered to 3 × kilograms × %TBSA.

MAINTENANCE FLUIDS

Next, give ½ NS at maintenance level. After the first 24 hours, titrate fluids to maintain urine output of 0.5 cc per hour. Give albumin (SPA) in the fourth 8-hr period *(0.1 × kilograms × %TBSA).*

NOTE: SPA is a 25% solution. If the institution stocks only Plasmanate (a 5% colloid solution), the calculation for colloid administration is 0.5 ml × kilograms 3 %TBSA.

MEDICATIONS

Topical Antibiotics

Silver sulfadiazine (Silvadene) or silver-impregnated dressing on body; bacitracin-polymyxin B (Polysporin) on face

Mycostatin (nystatin) 200,000 U PO/NGT q8h *(to inhibit bacterial transorption)*

Lactinex 1 g PO/NGT q6h

Tetanus toxoid 0.5 ml IM

HyperTet 250 U IM *(for older patient and/or if patient has no history of immunization)*

Omeprazole 20 mg qd PO/NGT. If no enteral access, 40 mg q12h IV. *(Use omeprazole for >20% burn.)*

MVI 10 ml IV qd

Folate 1 mg PO/NGT/IV qd

$MgSO_4$ 500 mg qw *(if >50% burn)*

Pain Medications

Dilaudid 2 mg IV q4h

MSO_4 8 mg IV q4h

Other Agents

Vitamin C 1000 mg PO/NGT/IV q6h

Znso4 220 mg PO/NGT tid

Selenium 50 mg PO/NGT bid

Vitamin E 400 U PO q6h

Beta carotene 25,000 U PO q12h

Heparin 7500 U SQ q8h, or Lovenox 40 mg q12h

Metamucil 1 tbsp PO/NGT bid

Codeine 30 mg PO q6h prn for diarrhea

ADDITIONAL ORDERS

If the patient has an eye burn:
>   Polysporin ophthalmic solution (formulation and strength carried by the institution's pharmacy)

If the patient has a pulmonary injury:
>   Aminophyline (6.0 mg/kg IV load, then 0.5 mg/kg/hr IV)
>   Ventolin (0.5 mg in 2 ml NS via nebulizer q4h and prn)
>   Heparin 4000 U (mix with Ventolin nebulizer in the 2 ml NS) will help to decrease pulmonary casts.
>   *(Consider bronchoscopic evaluation.)*

If the patient has no pulmonary injury:
>   Oxygen per nasal cannula or high-humidity face mask
>   Chest physical therapy

If the patient has sustained electrical injury:
>   Complete spine series *(Be sure to visualize C7-T1.)*
>   Long bone radiographic film series
>   Urine myoglobin and hemoglobin assay
>   Dopamine, renal dose, 1-4 μg/kg/hr IV

If the patient is elderly (optional):
>   Dopamine, renal dose, 1-4 μg/kg/hr IV

EXTRA ORDERS

NGT to LCWS flush q2h with 30 ml NS
Daily weight measurement
Bed in 20-degree semi-Fowler position
Elevate extremities
Foot cradle, splints
Foot pumps
Abduct shoulders
Foley to gravity
Pressure sore precautions
No pillow for a head/neck burn

VENTILATOR SETTINGS AND PEEP

Preferred ventilator: VDR$_4$

    Initial settings

        Oscillatory rate 600 breaths/min

        PIP 30-35 cm H$_2$O

        2-sec inspiration

        2-sec expiration

If the institution does not have this equipment available, these settings are used. Burn patients require increased respiratory rate and decreased tidal volume, because contraction from the burn limits chest expansion. Therefore start at AC 15-20, VT 5-10 ml/kg. Check an ABG in 30 minutes and make adjustments accordingly.

ABG *(30 min after the patient is placed on the ventilator; make changes accordingly)*

ABG/carboxyhemoglobin *(on admission and prn)*

ECG *(on admission and prn)*

CXR *(on admission; we usually obtain one on M and F, and prn. A CXR is obtained qd for patients receiving ventilatory support; assess for infiltrate, tube placement, pneumothorax.)*

LABORATORY TESTS

CBC *(on admission and W)*

SMA-12 *(on admission and M)*

SMA-7 *(on admission and M-W-F and prn)*

PT/PT *(on admission and prn)*

Sputum C&S *(on admission and qd and prn)*

Ca, Mg, Phos *(on admission and biweekly)*

H&H/electrolytes *(q8h until the patient is stable and then prn)*

Finger-stick blood glucose *(on admission and tid and prn)*

Urine 24-hr electrolytes *(on admission)*

HIV/EtOH/urine drug screen *(on admission)*
B-HCG *(if patient is female)*
Sickle cell panel *(if patient is black)*
Eschar BX (prn)
Albumin, prealbumin, transferrin *(qw [on M])*

CONSULTATIONS

OT/PT
Nutrition

OTHER CONSULTATIONS *(prn)*

(Consent is required for HIV testing, placing central lines, grafting, blood transfusions.)

CRITICAL CARE: ORGANIZATION FOR NOTES AND PRESENTATION
SHORT HISTORY

"This is Mr. X, a 25-year-old black male postburn day 3 s/p 50% TBSA burns after falling asleep while smoking in bed. He is also POD 2 from wound debridement and STSG to chest, along with application of pigskin to the remainder of the burned area."

T_{MAX}, INPUT/OUTPUT

NEUROLOGIC

Awake/alert, oriented ×3, GCS
Sedated, agent, rate
Paralysis, agent, rate
Focal vs. nonfocal

PULMONARY

Examination
Secretions
Ventilator settings
    AC vs. SIMV vs. CPAP/rate/pressure
    Spontaneous rate/Vt/FIO_2/PEEP/pressure support
    ABG
    CXR evaluation

CV/HEMODYNAMIC

Pulse, BP, patient on any pressors (dopamine, dobutamine)
Swan-Ganz catheter parameters
PAP/wedge/CO/SVR/SVO_2 or MVO_2
Electrolytes, anion gap, lactate
O_2 delivery, content

GI/NUTRITION

Examination
Obstruction series (if done)
Drainage output (if any)
BEE, calories needed, goal, plan to achieve that goal
    *(Note the location of the feeding catheter. Feedings to the stomach
    may increase tonicity first, followed by increased volume. Feedings
    to the small bowel increase volume first, then tonicity [to prevent
    diarrhea].)*
Feedings: name, strength, rate, route, nutritional parameters,
    UUN *(to compute nitrogen balance)*, transferrin, prealbumin,
    albumin

RENAL

Urine output (ml/kg/hr); minimum required is 0.5 ml/kg/hr
BUN/Cr or FENa if the UO is low

INFECTIOUS DISEASE/SEPSIS

WBC, blood and other cultures; site of focality; antibiotics (include day number)

ENDOCRINE

Function tests; LFTs; fingersticks; steroids

HEMATOLOGY/ONCOLOGY

Hb, platelet count, PT/PTT, coagulopathy studies *(if indicated)* SMA-7

SKIN

Percentage of burn, treatments, percentage take of graft *(may be brought up earlier in burn unit presentation)*
Pressure sore

EXTREMITIES

PT/OT treatment, progress

WHAT HAPPENS NEXT: THE PLAN
Debridement and Coverage

In general, the nonviable tissue is excised and the wound covered as soon as possible. Options for initial coverage include skin grafting, allograft, pigskin, cultured epithelial autograft (CEA), Alloderm with split-thickness skin grafts (STSG), and Integra.[13] (This subject is covered in more detail in Chapter 5.)

PREOPERATIVE EVALUATION

Vital signs
Procedure, indications
Laboratory tests

Type and crossmatch or screen for PRBCs *(This should be done at least 24 hours before surgery to allow the blood bank to obtain compatible blood when antibodies are present.)*

(Blood loss with debridement is now less of an issue because of the use of epinephrine/saline solution infiltration before debridement and skin harvesting from donor sites.)

CXR, ECG

Informed consent signed and on chart

OR notified; anesthesia team notified

REPEAT EXCISIONS AND GRAFTS

The ultimate goal of burn treatment is to close the wound as soon as possible, allowing the skin to heal spontaneously, or to use skin grafting to provide permanent coverage of the wound.

Rapid removal of the burn wound eliminates a source of tissue breakdown products, bacteria, and cytokine activation. This allows the patient to stabilize more quickly and results in a more desirable cosmetic and functional result.

Patients with large burn injuries may not have enough uninvolved skin to provide an adequate amount of donor skin. This should not delay excision of the burn wound, because other wound coverings are available. Excised surfaces may be covered temporarily with Integra, porcine xenograft, cadaver allograft, or Biobrane (in that order of desirability). Skin biopsies can be sent to allow cultured epithelial autograft.

SPECIAL AREAS OF BURN INJURY
Face

Suprathel has worked nicely on our patients with facial burns and has decreased formation of crusting. Burns on the face can also do well with daily application of bacitracin or another triple-antibiotic ointment. Patients with facial burns or a significant mechanism should have an ultraviolet light test for corneal abrasions; an ophthalmologic evaluation is indicated. Ears can be treated with mafenide only; this agent may decrease the incidence of chondritis and the risk of pressure necrosis. If the ears are to be wrapped, padding is carefully placed behind them to prevent pressure injury.[14]

Extremities

All burned extremities should be dressed with silver sulfadiazine (Silvadene) or silver-impregnated dressings. SurgiNet (expandable fishnet) over 4×4 sterile dressings works well. The extremities should be kept elevated. Hand burns can usually be cared for on an outpatient basis. Functional, vascular, and neurologic assessment should be documented. Digits should be maintained in a straight position and wrapped individually. Again, 4×4s with fishnet dressings work well. These patients should be seen the next day in the burn office. Close follow-up is crucial to the care of these patients. Early intervention with an occupational therapist is beneficial.

ALLIED HEALTH PRACTITIONERS: PART OF THE TEAM

Management of a burn patient is a multidisciplinary team effort and extends from the time of injury to completion of rehabilitation—that is, possibly years. All practitioners are important members of this team.

Occupational Therapists

Occupational therapists focus on the functions of the hand involving activities of daily living and on scar control. Modalities of therapy include splinting for immobilization and positioning, as well as any devices for patient mobilization and those that help patients adapt to their surroundings and abilities.

Physical Therapists

Physical therapists focus on burn patients' general mobility and the mobility of their extremities. Modalities include therapy, splinting, and adaptation devices. Spandex compression garments are cus-tom-fit to each patient. They compress the burned area in an effort to flatten and soften scar tissue as it matures. Inserts are sometimes placed within the spandex pressure garments to direct more pressure to areas that are difficult to compress with garments alone.

Dietitians

Dietitians focus on the nutrition status of burn patients, helping them to compensate for the tremendous metabolic needs associated with recovery (see Chapter 6). Nutrition is a crucial issue in these patients, because they need adequate substrates to heal their wounds and manage the endocrine and metabolic stresses. Dietitians can cal-culate the caloric requirements and monitor a patient's dietary and weight trends. They also understand the myriad enteral and peren-teral formulas that may benefit a patient.[15,16]

OTHER ISSUES

In our unit, central venous pressure (CVP) catheters are changed ev-ery 3 days. The first two CVP changes are over a wire. The third is a new stick. This pattern is then repeated (i.e., new stick, change over wire, change over wire; new stick, change over wire, change over wire). In our institution, this has significantly decreased the incidence of infection and thrombosis.

Intravenous antibiotics are given, guided by culture data and clinical evaluation. Clinical evaluation is needed to assess distinction between colonization and infection. Prophylactic antibiotic therapy is not used; this helps to prevent the appearance of more resistant organisms.

Often, burn patients have a mild fever secondary to their hyper-metabolic state. Therefore the threshold for fever workup, culturing, and treatment is 39° C (102° F) in most cases.[17,18]

The choice of bed is covered in greater detail in Chapter 8. Generally, the goal is to decrease the amount of sheering forces.

Some beds can help in pulmonary toilet, facilitating access to the patient for rotation and percussion therapy.

STEP-DOWN BURN CARE

Many patients are sent to a general hospital unit after the critical portion of their hospital course has been accomplished. Their intensive occupational therapy, physical therapy, and nutritional support continue.

Rehabilitation

The rehabilitation process that was started in the burn unit continues. Some patients need to go to a designated rehabilitation facility, whereas others may continue their therapy on an outpatient basis.

Preparing for Discharge to Home

The goal of therapy is to help the patient return home and resume his or her occupation or activities in the best functional condition possible. Modifications in the home situation are sometimes necessary. This can range from care issues to physical changes in the residence. Social workers and case managers are important resources in this aspect of care.[19] Some patients find pastoral care to be helpful.[20]

Psychiatric Care

Many burn patients have significant emotional trauma and stress involving physical self-image and possible loss of loved ones, home, and possessions from the burn incident. Emotional and psychological support are very important to a patient's outcome, rehabilitation, and adaptation. A psychiatrist can help the family or a significant other cope with the aftermath of a serious burn injury. There are self-help organizations and support groups for burn patients that address social, functional, and occupational concerns.[21]

Psychiatric consultation in the acute phase of a burn injury is as important as it is in follow-up care, after the patient is discharged.

Members of the burn team should understand that even relatively minor burn injuries can have a major psychological impact on the patient and family. They should not hesitate to recommend psychiatric evaluation and support.

REFERENCES

1. Advanced Trauma Life Support, ed 8. Chicago: American College of Surgeons, 2008.
2. Cupera J, Mannová J, Rihová H, et al. Quality of prehospital management of patients with burn injuries—a retrospective study. Acta Chir Plast 44:59-62, 2002.
3. Sheridan RL, Petras L, Basha G, et al. Planimetry study of the percent of body surface represented by the hand and palm. Sizing irregular burns is more accurately done with the palm. J Burn Care Rehabil 16:605-606, 1995.
4. Greenhalgh DG. Burn resuscitation: the results of the ISBI/ABA survey. Burns 36:176-182, 2010.
5. McBeth PB, Sass K, Nickerson D, et al. A necessary evil? Intra-abdominal hypertension complicating burn patient resuscitation. J Trauma Manag Outcomes 8:12, 2014.
6. Strang SG, Van Lieshout EM, Breederveld RS, et al. A systematic review on intra-abdominal pressure in severely burned patients. Burns 40:9-16, 2014.
7. Cancio LC. Initial assessment and fluid resuscitation of burn patients. Surg Clin North Am 94:741-754, 2014.
8. Navickis RJ, Greenhalgh DG, Wilkes MM. Albumin in burn shock resuscitation: a meta-analysis of controlled clinical studies. J Burn Care Res 2014 Nov 25. [Epub ahead of print]
9. Sheridan RL, Chang P. Acute burn procedures. Surg Clin North Am 94:755-764, 2014.
10. Fagan SP, Bilodeau ML, Goverman J. Burn intensive care. Surg Clin North Am 94:765-779, 2014.
11. Pruitt BA Jr. Reflection: evolution of the field over seven decades. Surg Clin North Am 94:721-740, 2014.
12. Sheridan RL, Greenhalgh D. Special problems in burns. Surg Clin North Am 94:781-791, 2014.
13. Deitch EA. A policy of early excision and grafting in elderly burn patients shortens the hospital stay and improves survival. Burns Incl Therml Inj 12:109-114, 1985.
14. Stanton RA, Billmire DA. Skin resurfacing for the burned patient. Clin Plast Surg 29(1):29-51, 2002.

15. LeVoyer T, Cioffi WG Jr, Pratt L, et al. Alterations in intestinal permeability after thermal injury. Arch Surg 127:26-29, 1992.
16. Sefton EJ, Boulton-Jones JR, Anderton D, et al. Enteral feeding in patients with major burn injury: the use of nasojejunal feeding after the failure of nasogastric feeding. Burns 28:386-390, 2002.
17. Sheridan RL, Weber JM, Pasternack MS, et al. Antibiotic prophylaxis for group A streptococcal burn wound infection is not necessary. J Trauma 51:352-355, 2001.
18. Thompson JT, Meredith JW, Molnar JA. The effect of burn nursing units on burn wound infections. J Burn Care Rehabil 23:281-286, 2002.
19. Oster C, Kildal M, Ekselius L. Return to work after burn injury: burn-injured individuals' perception of barriers and facilitators. J Burn Care Res 31:540-550, 2010.
20. Hultman CS, Saou MA, Roach ST, et al. To heal and restore broken bodies: a retrospective, descriptive study of the role and impact of pastoral care in the treatment of patients with burn injury. Ann Plast Surg 72:289-294, 2014.
21. Williams RM, Patterson DR, Schwenn C, et al. Evaluation of a peer consultation program for burn inpatients. 2000 ABA paper. J Burn Care Rehabil 23:449-453, 2002.

4 Admissions and Follow-up Care

KEY POINTS

- The American Burn Association has set guidelines for burn specialists.

- The burn team provides supportive care for burn patients.

- Patients with smaller burns may need to be admitted and treated until they are comfortable.

- Pain control is an important part of burn care.

- Many smaller burns can be treated effectively in an outpatient setting.

- Palliative care can be an asset to help families of burn patients at the end of life.

The American Burn Association has adopted criteria for evaluation by a burn unit[1]:

- Partial-thickness burns of greater than 10% of the body surface area (BSA)
- Burns that involve the face, hands, feet, genitalia, perineum, or major joints
- Third-degree burns in any age group
- Electrical burns, including lightning injury

- Chemical burns
- Inhalation injury
- Burn injury in patients with preexisting medical disorders that could complicate management, prolong recovery, or affect mortality
- Any patient with burns and concomitant trauma (such as fractures), in whom the burn injury poses the greatest risk of morbidity or mortality. In such cases, if the trauma poses the greater immediate risk, the patient may be initially stabilized in a trauma center before being transferred to a burn unit. Physician judgment will be necessary and should be in concert with the regional medical control plan and triage protocols.
- Burned children in hospitals that do not have qualified personnel or equipment for the care of children
- Burn injury in patients who will require special social, emotional, or rehabilitation care

Patients who meet any of these criteria should be seen by burn specialists. Burn units have specially trained personnel and are often unique physical units with access to various resources (such as therapy and social work) for treating a variety of injuries and other related problems.[2-5]

Often emergency medicine physicians will choose to transfer these patients to the burn unit. Our facility will always agree to see a burn patient in transfer. All transfer phone calls go directly to the burn attending physician. Many of these patients can be followed in the office, but the referring facility prefers to transfer them. These patients are usually transferred to the emergency department for evaluation, and many can be discharged and given instructions to follow up in the office.[6]

OTHER INDICATIONS FOR ADMISSION TO THE BURN UNIT

Patients are admitted to the hospital burn service for many reasons. Some with smaller burns need to be admitted. Most burns are not catastrophic injuries that necessitate intubation and direct admission to the unit. Often patients have confounding issues that warrant admission under the burn service.

One reason to admit a patient is to monitor the airway. If a patient has a history of exposure to smoke in an enclosed space but does not have stridor, it may be prudent to watch the airway overnight for signs of edema. Rarely, the patient will need to be intubated. The presence of facial burns can cause edema of the periorbital tissue with closure of the eyes because of the rich blood supply in this area. Edema usually resolves within 24 hours, but for such patients who live alone, the presence of edema can lead to a dangerous situation.

Patients who have bilateral hand burns may have difficulty with activities of daily living. They can be admitted, and dressing changes can be placed. These patients are seen by an occupational therapist.

Acute burns initially cause pain and anxiety, especially on the first day. Many patients with smaller burns require intravenous medication for comfort. This can be quickly transitioned to oral analgesics.

Some patients with smaller burns need to be admitted because their residence is uninhabitable from the fire or because they are homeless. Case managers and social workers are invaluable in these situations. Patients who burned themselves often need to be admitted for psychiatric evaluation. These patients are difficult to discharge and many times cannot go to a psychiatric hospital with open wounds.

OUTPATIENT AND FOLLOW-UP CARE

Most patients with burns can be seen in an outpatient setting. At our institution, we see outpatients in the office three afternoons a week. Patients with larger burns requiring more office time are seen in the hospital's wound care area. Some patients can be referred to an occupational therapist and have their scars managed in the office setting.[7] Many with smaller, full-thickness burns can have graft procedures as outpatients and can follow up in the office.[8] Insurance companies will sometimes deny admission for inpatient skin grafting; if pain is manageable with oral analgesics, admission is often not needed.

Most of our patients are seen weekly for 2 to 4 weeks, until their wounds heal and they can resume their preinjury lifestyle. A small number of patients are followed for a longer time. Scarring is one reason for a longer follow-up. Wounds that have been grafted or take longer than 3 weeks to heal can develop hypertrophic scarring. The wound is elevated within the boundaries of the scar. It is not a keloid. These scars develop because too much epithelium is produced. The healed skin may undergo remodeling for up to 2 years. The use of pressure garments and silicone have been the mainstay of therapy. The garments are worn 23 hours a day for up to 2 years. Silicone may help to hydrate tissues and can be used under the garments or alone.[9-11]

Recently we have used a carbon dioxide laser for scar revision. The laser is biphasic with a deep component to "drill" deep into the scar and break up the collagen. This loosens and flattens the scar, similar to placing skin through a mesher. A superficial component is fractionally ablative and blends the skin with the other tissues. This modality can be used on mature scars and facilitates remodeling.[12] Our most important finding is that it releases some of the associated contracture related to the scar. These effects can be immediate; many patients state at the time of the procedure that their joints move better. Therapy should be reinitiated after laser scar revision, along with the use of pressure garments and silicone dressings.

Pain control is another reason patients continue to receive outpatient care. Some have true lingering pain and need medications to help them continue therapy. Others have an addictive personality and will continue to seek narcotics. All attempts should be made to wean patients from narcotics. Instructing patients that antiinflammatory medications will be more beneficial after the wound closes sometimes eases the transition. Those who continue to need narcotics can be given methadone. Patients should also be referred to a pain service.

Contractures respond well to excision and skin grafting or Z-plasty. Patients with larger affected areas may need to be referred to the plastic surgery service for tissue transfer or placement of tissue expanders. Bald areas on the head after electrical injuries respond well to tissue transfers after placement of tissue expanders.[13-15]

When patients are evaluated in the office to determine whether they can return to work, signs of posttraumatic stress need to be noted. This is common in patients who have had a work-related injury. Usually, work is considered a safe place, and a patient may feel anxious about returning to this environment. Nightmares and difficulty sleeping (tossing and turning in bed) are common symptoms of posttraumatic stress. Usually, the patient's significant other is asked about these occurrences, because they are awakened by them. Sertraline (Zoloft) can be given as a pharmacologic treatment. The patient is informed that it can take 2 weeks to feel the effects of this medication. It is also beneficial for the patient to see a psychiatrist or psychologist well versed in posttraumatic stress issues. Fortunately, the effects of posttraumatic stress will usually gradually fade. Social workers and case managers can also facilitate the transition back to work.[16,17]

PALLIATIVE CARE

Unfortunately, not all patients will survive their stay in the burn unit. Extensive metabolic stresses are placed on the body. Many patients with large burns have an elevated heart rate for weeks. Mortality increases in patients 50 years of age and older, because the body cannot keep up with the metabolic demands. Most families will initially want everything possible to be done to help the patient. As the patient develops more system failures, the palliative care service can be beneficial. They can help the family make decisions when the patient has no chance of survival. Many families do not know how to cope with the grief and feelings of guilt that can occur with end-of-life decisions. The palliative care service also can help in this regard.

REFERENCES

1. American Burn Association. Committee on Trauma, American College of Surgeons. Resources for optimal care of the injured patient 2014. Guidelines for trauma centers caring for burn patients. Chicago: The Burn Association, 2014.
2. Sheridan RL, Greenhalgh D. Special problems in burns. Surg Clin North Am 94:781-791, 2014.
3. Fagan SP, Bilodeau ML, Goverman J. Burn intensive care. Surg Clin North Am 94:765-779, 2014.
4. Pruitt BA Jr. Reflection: evolution of the field over seven decades. Surg Clin North Am 94:721-740, 2014.
5. Sheridan RL, Chang P. Acute burn procedures. Surg Clin North Am 94:755-764, 2014.
6. Cancio LC. Initial assessment and fluid resuscitation of burn patients. Surg Clin North Am 94:741-754, 2014.
7. Atiyeh B, Janom HH. Physical rehabilitation of pediatric burns. Ann Burns Fire Disasters 27:37-43, 2014.
8. Warner PM, Coffee TL, Yowler CJ. Outpatient burn management. Surg Clin North Am 94:879-892, 2014.
9. Yagmur C, Akaishi S, Ogawa R, et al. Mechanical receptor-related mechanisms in scar management: a review and hypothesis. Plast Reconstr Surg 126:426-434, 2010.
10. Atiyeh BS, El Khatib AM, Dibo SA. Pressure garment therapy (PGT) of burn scars: evidence-based efficacy. Ann Burns Fire Disasters 26:205-212, 2013.
11. Bloemen MC, van der Veer WM, Ulrich MM, et al. Prevention and curative management of hypertrophic scar formation. Burns 35:463-475, 2009.
12. Hultman CS, Friedstat JS, Edkins RE, et al. Laser resurfacing and remodeling of hypertrophic burn scars: the results of a large, prospective, before-after cohort study, with long-term follow-up. Ann Surg 260:519-529; discussion 529-532, 2014.
13. Wainwright DJ. Burn reconstruction: the problems, the techniques, and the applications. Clin Plast Surg 36:687-700, 2009.
14. MacLennan SE, Corcoran JF, Neale HW. Tissue expansion in head and neck burn reconstruction. Clin Plast Surg 27:121-132, 2000.
15. Furnas H, Lineaweaver WC, Alpert BS, et al. Scalp reconstruction by microvascular free tissue transfer. Ann Plast Surg 24:431-444, 1990.
16. Oster C, Kildal M, Ekselius L. Return to work after burn injury: burn-injured individuals' perception of barriers and facilitators. J Burn Care Res 31:540-550, 2010.
17. Gullick JG, Taggart SB, Johnston RA, et al. The trauma bubble: patient and family experience of serious burn injury. J Burn Care Res 35:e413-e427, 2014.

5 Wound Care, Use of Antibiotics, and Control of Burn Wound Sepsis

KEY POINTS

- Wounds are a source of infection in burn patients.
- Third-degree burns should be excised in the first week.
- Many topical antibiotics are available for use.
- Systemic antibiotics are used for burn wound sepsis and pneumonias.

The rate of survival in burn patients has improved considerably in the past few decades. As a result of continuous development in the treatment of burns, the LD_{50} (the burn size lethal to 50% of the population) for thermal injuries has risen from 42% body surface area (BSA) during the 1940s and 1950s to more than 90% BSA for young thermally injured patients.[1] This can be attributed to advances in resuscitation, nutritional support, pulmonary care, wound care, and infection control.[2] Sepsis is the leading cause of death in patients with large burns.[3,4] Seventy-five percent of all deaths after burn injury are related to infection. Ninety-one percent of patients dying with burn wound sepsis have positive bacterial or fungal cultures.[5]

In the 1940s early mortality of burn patients was usually caused by shock. After the Coconut Grove nightclub tragedy in Boston in

1942, in which 492 people died, aggressive resuscitation with fluid and electrolytes became standard practice.[6] Patients typically lived an average of 3 days, only to die from *Streptococcus* sepsis. In 1945 the use of penicillin, along with fluid and electrolyte management, became the standard of treatment. Patients then typically died 2 weeks later from penicillin-resistant *Staphylococcus*. Penicillin-resistant antibiotics were developed in the 1950s. Patients then succumbed to infection by gram-negative organisms. Infection with *Pseudomonas* organisms began to be seen in increasing numbers.[7] The organisms now found in patients range from the common nosocomial bacteria (e.g., *Staphylococcus*, beta-hemolytic *Streptococcus*, *Pseudomonas aeruginosa*, and *Escherichia coli*) to more exotic bacteria selected out by widespread antibiotic use, such as methicillin-resistant *S. aureus* (MRSA), *Klebsiella*, *Enterobacter*, *Proteus*, *Provodentia*, and *Serratia*.[8] *Acinetobacter* presentation also continues to increase and has proved costly in the burn unit population.[9-11] Fungal infection with such organisms such as *Candida albicans* is increasing. The incidence of nonalbicans *Candida* infection (especially *C. tropicalis* and *C. krusei*) is rising, compared with that of *C. albicans*. Nonalbicans infections are more severe in nature and associated with a higher mortality. This signifies a shift in fungal wound infection in burns from commensal organisms (e.g., *C. albicans*) to a more pathogenic nosocomial organism.[12] *Aspergillus* is also becoming more common and problematic.[13] Individual hospital units will notice a change in their common pathogens over time, and continued surveillance is essential.[14] Prevention continues to be a cornerstone of infection control.[15-18]

PATHOPHYSIOLOGY

With a burn injury, the normal skin barrier against bacteria is lost. This is combined with local release of cytokines, immunosuppressive factors, ischemia (with breakdown of normal tissue and circulating cellular components), wound maceration, high moisture content, and acidic pH. Later, endotoxins, exotoxins, and enzymes from microbes have local and systemic effects. This subsequently leads to hyper-metabolism and catabolism, eventually depleting energy stores and decreasing the body's resistance to infection.[19,20] Blood supply to the wound is usually compromised by the thermal injury, secondary to edema and thrombosis of the vasculature.

Microbes may descend through the eschar and enter the subeschar plane. Enzymes released by microorganisms and white blood cells (WBCs) cause lysis of denatured burn wound proteins. This provides more nutritional substrates for the bacteria. Bacterial growth can sometimes be held in check at the interface between the eschar and the viable tissue.

Topical administration of antibiotics is helpful to distribute the antimicrobial compound at the involved site.[15] Topical agents will not sterilize a burn wound. Their use is intended to control bacterial growth on the burn wound.[21-24]

Further breakdown of host defenses may tip the balance in favor of the bacteria advancing into the adjacent, healthy tissue. Hematologous spread follows invasion of bacteria into the viable tissues. The goals of treatment for a burn patient include the prevention of sepsis and the preservation of function and form.

The management of burn wounds is part of the overall treatment strategy. This includes many aspects of a patient's care. Resuscitation is important to ensure adequate cardiopulmonary function—essential for tissue perfusion and immunologic reserve for wound healing and prevention of burn sepsis. Cardiopulmonary function is also significant for nutrition, antibiotics, and oxygen transport to the tissues. Without cardiopulmonary function, the necessary materials cannot travel from where they are to where they are needed (e.g., intravenous antibiotics need to travel through the bloodstream to the infected area).

Advances in critical care have also contributed to the improvement in the management of burn patients. Our ability to monitor perfusion and fluid status in the resuscitative period and beyond has greatly improved. This can lead to early detection and intervention in cardiac function, systemic perfusion, or sepsis.

Improvements in the understanding and management of the nutritional needs of this unique population have resulted in better outcomes. Burn patients have very high metabolic needs, with an increase in the basic metabolic rate as high as 2 to 2.5 times the basal energy expenditure. The role of early enteric support has also been appreciated, which is seen as preservation of the integrity of the bowel lumen and subsequent prevention of translocation of bacteria and cytokines across the bowel wall. This may decrease susceptibility to infection.[25] The support of the immune system is also important, because profound immunosuppression usually follows major injury.[5,26,27]

Decreasing the translocation of bacteria, cytokines, and endotoxins may help to decrease the manifestations of systemic infection. The intent is not to sterilize the bowel per se, but to decrease the amount of bacteria and toxins that travel across the bowel wall. Support of the mucosa is important, as mentioned earlier. Indications for this therapy are burns greater than 20% total burned surface area (TBSA).

Control of translocation may offer an additional local benefit in the pulmonary tissue (in light of the lymphatic flow drawing from the peritoneal cavity toward the diaphragm), where translocated bacteria and toxins can compound the insults of smoke inhalation and respiratory depression that contribute to increased rates of pulmonary infection. Pneumonia is a well-known and significant complication in this patient population.

The isolation of burn patients is associated with a decreased incidence of gram-negative sepsis and improved survival.[28]

COMMON PATHOGENS

Certain bacteria typically are found in burn wounds. Principally, gram-positive bacteria isolated from burn wounds are Staphylococci and beta-hemolytic Streptococci. The most common gram-negative bacteria are *P. aeruginosa* and *E. coli*. Other gram-negative organisms seen include *Klebsiella*, *Enterobacter*, *Proteus*, *Provodentia*, and *Serratia*. Fungi, especially *C. albicans*, are also seen.[8]

The most common causative organisms of burn sepsis are gram-negative bacilli. These include *E. coli*, *Klebsiella*, *Enterobacter*, *Proteus*, *Providencia*, *Serratia marcescens*, and *P. aeruginosa*. These are frequently found to be nosocomial organisms that may be resistant to conventional antibiotic therapy. *S. aureus* is another significant cause of infection in burn patients. MRSA may also arise in some burn units.[8]

INITIAL MANAGEMENT OF THE WOUND

Louis Pasteur stated, "The germ is nothing, it is the terrain in which it grows which is everything."[29] An eschar is an excellent culture medium. This avascular space will eventually become colonized with bacteria. It may become colonized despite the application of topical antibiotics. Our institution uses a Collagenase/Polysporin powder. This provides antibiotic protection and will help to loosen the eschar for eventual debridement.

The cornerstone of burn wound care is prompt excision of necrotic tissue and closure of the wounds that are healing slowly with skin grafts or biologic dressings. Host resistance can now be adequately protected and the possibility of wound contamination minimized.[15] Early wound closure may be associated with lower rates of infection and mortality.[30,31] Our institution will perform an escharectomy for full-thickness burns on days 0 to 5. Skin grafts for partial-thickness burns are performed on or approximately on day 18. These guidelines are followed, with consideration for the clinical evaluation, coloration, and consistency of the wound and the patient's condition. Excised eschar is sent for culture and sensitivities. A wound biopsy is performed in the first week. Biopsies are not typically performed after 2 weeks.

In patients with large areas of unequivocal full-thickness burns, direct excision to fascia is the procedure of choice. In patients with mixed deep-dermal and full-thickness injuries, and in those in whom the exact area of full-thickness burn is difficult to determine, sequential eschar excisions are performed.

Larger burns may require staged excision and often allograft or Integra for closure. Fresh donor sites are also at risk for infection. Superficial second-degree burns that are not excised need protection. A variety of modalities can now be used to cover the burn. As stated previously, early excision and coverage lowers the risk of infection, decreases metabolic work, and results in better outcomes.

Split-thickness skin grafts can be used to cover full-thickness burns. Such grafts use the patient's own tissue and are a mainstay of treatment. One disadvantage is that the donor site is now another wound that needs to heal. If a patient has massive wounds, harvesting additional skin may not be an option. The patient may have "run out of skin" (e.g., a patient with a 60% burn has only 40% of the skin left). We will graft partial thickness, because the metabolic state slows the 2-week usual healing time. Harvested areas can usually be reused after they are healed in 2 to 3 weeks.

Not all of the remaining skin can be used (e.g., harvesting from the face); the patient needs an alternative form of coverage for the debrided wound.

Temporary coverage is often a viable alternative. Cadaver skin and pigskin can be used in this manner. Such a graft will eventually slough, but it will buy time until the body is less hypermetabolic and more of the patient's own skin can be used.

Permanent coverage using various commercial modalities is now possible. Alloderm is a cultured, processed dermis that aids in graft take and serves as a biologic scaffold for normal tissue remodeling.

The meshed Alloderm is placed on the burn wound, and a skin graft is placed on top of the Alloderm. Histologically, the dermis does not show that the patient has been burned. However, no sweat glands or hair follicles are seen. We use this modality in large burn wounds.

Integra is another modality currently in use. This product, billed as "skin off the shelf," is made from bovine connective tissue. Strips of Integra are placed on the wound as a skin graft would be. We have used this modality on significant-size wounds to achieve coverage in one procedure. This modality has been especially effective on wounds across joints, with improved range of motion. The areas covered with Integra form a neodermis and must be grafted after 3 to 4 weeks to heal.

Although most grafts take in the first few days after a burn injury, complete closure seldom occurs. Protection from infection is required.

Protection from infection includes recognizing personnel and family as potential sources of contamination. Isolation measures are necessary, such as gowning of caregivers and the use of patient-specific items. The importance of hand-washing must be stressed.

INFECTED WOUNDS

Infected wounds are a serious problem in burn patients. Infection does not allow the burn to heal. Infection delays epidermal maturation and leads to additional scar tissue formation.[32] Infection continues to stimulate the patient's hypermetabolic state. Treatment includes clysis, as guided by biopsy. *Clysis* is a procedure in which a substance—in this case, antibiotics—is injected under the plane of tissue. It can be used to separate the skin layer from the underlying tissue and to control operative blood loss. For example, clysis can be performed using one ampule of epinephrine mixed with 1 L of normal saline solution. Parenteral antibiotics are indicated when wound biopsies show bacterial counts of greater than 1×10^5 per cubic centimeter of tissue. This is also the point at which healing of the wound is compromised. Parenteral antibiotics are not usually given until just before surgery or for burn wound infection.[33-35]

PREOPERATIVE PARENTERAL ANTIBIOTICS

Preoperative parenteral antibiotics are selected against the organism found in the biopsy.[30] These are given before the operation because of the bacteremia produced at the time of the operation.[36] Parenteral antibiotics should cover *P. aeruginosa* and staphylococci.[37] Choices of antibiotics include vancomycin and amikacin, nafcillin and an aminoglycoside, or antipseudomonal penicillin and an aminoglycoside. Other treatments include a cephalosporin and an aminoglycoside or vancomycin and an aminoglycoside.[8] Amikacin is becoming a preferred substitution for aminoglycosides. Imipenem has been shown to be very useful, especially postoperatively, as guided by culture data.

TETANUS PROPHYLAXIS

A burn is an open wound. In our institution, standard practice is to administer tetanus immune globulin prophylactically for patients who have not had such prophylaxis in the past 5 years.

TOPICAL ANTIBIOTICS

Topical antibiotics control microbiologic invasion of open wounds much more effectively than systemic antibiotics.[21,22,24] The choice of a topical antibiotic should follow the general rules outlined previously. They are intended to limit colonization and to control growth of pathologic organisms. Topical antibiotics may decrease cytokines and chemical mediators. They may act by changing the chemical makeup of the burn wound milieu rather than through the actual bacteriostatic or bactericidal effect. Some institutions change the topical antibiotics every 7 days to increase the effectiveness and to decrease the possibility of selecting out resistant strains of pathogens. The use of the topical antibiotic is guided first empirically, or by the resident flora of the individual burn unit. Patients who arrive after being in an institution should be noted (e.g., nursing home residents with a nosocomial infection who sustain burn injury and are admitted to the burn unit).[38]

We recommend applying a topical agent to the dressing, which is then placed on the wound. This is more comfortable for the patient and prevents contamination of the topical agent's receptacle by contact with the patient's burned skin.

If the bacterial load of the wound is a concern after a skin graft has been placed, topical antibiotics are applied. Usually, this consists of topical Sulfamylon 5% solution (NB: not the 12% cream) or silver nitrate.

Dressings impregnated with silver (Acticoat or Mepilex Ag) can also be useful in wounds in which a high bacterial load is suspected.

COLLAGENASE/POLYSPORIN POWDER   This powder is used less frequently. In selected cases, Collagenase/Polysporin powder can be effective, well tolerated, and in keeping with the total management plan of the patient (i.e., removal of dead tissue/culture medium eschar). This modality also provides antimicrobial coverage.[23]

SILVER SULFADIAZINE (SILVADENE)   Silver sulfadiazine is the most commonly used topical antibiotic. It is used extensively for outpatient and inpatient treatment. It has excellent broad-spectrum coverage and is effective against *Candida*. This agent can be used with or without a dressing and is painless and easy to apply. Drawbacks include leukopenia and poor eschar penetration. Our institution uses it as a first-line outpatient and inpatient topical antibiotic.

BETADINE, A 10% OINTMENT OF POVIDONE-IODINE   Povidone-iodine ointment has broad antimicrobial properties. Its main active ingredient is iodine. It can be used on open or closed wounds. The best antimicrobial activity is seen when it is administered every 6 hours. It can produce pain, immune depression, kidney dysfunction, and thyroid dysfunction. This modality should not be used in children and pregnant women because of the potential for iodine toxicity. The main use at this time is to prepare a wound for excision by drawing fluid from it, making the surface hard, mechanically allowing an easier excision.

SILVER NITRATE, AgNO₃ 0.5% SOLUTION   Silver nitrate is a broad-spectrum bacteriostatic topical agent that is painless on application. It has limited eschar penetration (similar to Silvadene), because the silver is quickly bound to the body's natural chemical compounds, such as chloride. It is light sensitive, turning black on contact with tissues and chloride-containing substances. The agent leaches NaCl from the tissue, so hyponatremia may become a problem. Monitoring of electrolytes is important. The agent can also cause methemoglobinemia, because the organisms will break down the compound from NO_3 to NO_2 form, which is absorbed by the patient. Bulky cotton dressings, thicker than 1 inch, are used. Soaks every 2 hours around the clock are needed, along with twice-daily dressing changes. Hypothermia is a concern with the use of silver nitrate because of its evaporative cooling effect. Burn patients must be kept warm. This agent is used only in specialized units.

MAFENIDE ACETATE (SULFAMYLON)   Mafenide acetate allows excellent penetration of full-thickness eschar. It is equal in efficacy to Silvadene against gram-negative organisms. It decreases bacterial counts and is easy to apply. It is especially effective against *Clostridia* and *Pseudomonas* organisms. It has a narrow spectrum of activity, mostly against gram-negative rods. Mafenide acetate does not affect *Candida*. It can cause metabolic acidosis, because it is a carbonic anhydrase inhibitor. Rarely, it can cause an aplastic crisis. Caution is needed when using it on a wound of greater than 70% TBSA because of the potential for metabolic acidosis. This modality causes pain to the patient when applied. A 5% solution is usually less painful than the 12% (hyperosmotic) cream.

GENTAMICIN   Gentamicin is an antibiotic that decreases wound colonization against *Pseudomonas*. Rapidly emerging resistant organisms sometimes prohibit its use. This drug is also not often used systemically because of the selection of resistant organisms in the wound. Amikacin is becoming a preferred substitution for the aminoglycosides.

NYSTATIN, MICONAZOLE TO CONTROL *CANDIDA* AND *PHYCOMYCETES* These antifungal agents are mixed with mafenide or sulfadiazine and applied topically to control *Candida*. Nystatin oral wash (swish) is used to control thrush, especially with concomitant antibacterial usage. This may assume more of a role in the future, because the use of wide-spectrum antibiotics is changing the flora found in burn units and burn wounds.

SILVER-IMPREGNATED DRESSINGS Numerous silver-based dressings are now available, such as Acticoat and Mepilex Ag. These dressings allow constant release of silver ions into the wound. The dressing can be changed every 3 to 5 days, depending on which is used. We also have found that a pseudoeschar is less likely to develop if an Ace wrap is placed over the dressing.

SYSTEMIC ANTIFUNGAL AGENTS

AMPHOTERICIN B Amphotericin B has long been used as a systemic antifungal agent. Dosing includes setting a goal dose (6 mg/kg), then working up to it. The usual starting dose is 0.25 to 0.50 mg/kg. The duration of therapy then depends on how long it takes to reach the goal dose. A test dose (1 mg in 100 ml) should be applied before therapy is started. The normal concentration of amphotericin B is 0.1 mg/ml. The drug has side effects that include fever, nausea, vomiting, and hypokalemia.

DIFLUCAN Fluconazole (Diflucan) is a well-used systemic antifungal agent. It is effective and does not have the unique dosing necessary for or the profound side effects of amphotericin. This agent may have an increasing role in the near future. It is our institution's first-line parenteral antifungal agent. Other systemic antifungal agents will soon be available and should help to address the increasing incidence of fungal infection.

A UNIQUE POPULATION

Burn patients are unique in many ways. The metabolic stress, pathophysiology, and cutaneous wound of a burn injury all have systemic effects. The psychologic aspects of self-image and the physiologic factors (e.g., range of motion and mobility) are distinct from those encountered in other patient populations.

Basic surgical principles are of paramount importance. Debridement of tissue, control of infection, nutritional and physiologic support, and prevention of sepsis may be magnified in burn patients. The role of the burn surgeon is to attempt to control the many variables to achieve the best possible outcome.[39]

Most wounds will become contaminated in a few days; therefore the "golden period" for excision therapy is 5 to 7 days. After this time, patients undergoing excision will be subjected to bacteremia during excision of the eschar. Prophylactic antibiotics are given to prevent this problem.

Antibiotic therapy, guided by clinical evaluation and cultures, must be tailored to each patient.[40]

REFERENCES

1. Fagan SP, Bilodeau ML, Goverman J. Burn intensive care. Surg Clin North Am 94:765-779, 2014.
2. Pruitt BA Jr. Reflection: evolution of the field over seven decades. Surg Clin North Am 94:721-740, 2014.
3. Edwards-Jones V, Greenwood JE; Manchester Burns Research Group. What's new in burn microbiology? James Laing Memorial Prize Essay 2000. Burns 29:15-24, 2003.
4. Williams FN, Herndon DN, Hawkins HK, et al. The leading causes of death after burn injury in a single pediatric burn center. Crit Care 13:R183, 2009.
5. Hansbrough JF. Burn wound sepsis. J Intensive Care Med 2:313-327, 1987.
6. Saffle JR. The 1942 fire at Boston's Coconut Grove nightclub. Am J Surg 166:581-591, 1993.
7. Krizek T. Local factors influencing incidence of wound sepsis. Symposium on antibiotic prophylaxis and therapy. Contemp Surg 10:45-50, 1977.

8. Lampe KF. Antimicrobial therapy and chemoprophylaxis of infectious diseases. In American Medical Association, ed. Drug Evaluations Annual, ed 7. Chicago: American Medical Association, 1991.

9. Siegel JD, Rhinehart E, Jackson M, et al; Healthcare Infection Control Practices Advisory Committee. Management of multidrug-resistant organisms in health care settings, 2006. Am J Infect Control 32:342-344, 2004.

10. Wilson SJ, Knipe CJ, Zieger MJ, et al. Direct costs of multidrug-resistant Acinetobacter baumannii in the burn unit of a public teaching hospital. Am J Infect Control 32:342-344, 2004.

11. Gootz TD, Marra A. Acinetobacter baumannii: an emerging multidrug-resistant threat. Expert Rev Anti Infect Ther 6:309-325, 2008.

12. Sarabahi S, Tiwari VK, Arora S, et al. Changing pattern of fungal infection in burn patients. Burns 38:520-528, 2012.

13. Murray CK, Loo FL, Hospenthal DR, et al. Incidence of systemic fungal infection and related mortality following severe burns. Burns 34:1108-1112, 2008.

14. Raz-Pasteur A, Hussein K, Finkelstein R, et al. Blood stream infections (BSI) in severe burn patients—early and late BSI: a 9-year study. Burns 39:636-642, 2013.

15. Mousa HA, al-Bader SM. Yeast infection of burns. Mycoses 44:147-149, 2001.

16. Lee HG, Jang J, Choi JE, et al. Blood stream infections in patients in the burn intensive care unit. Infect Chemother 45:194-201, 2013.

17. Struck MF, Gille J. Fungal infections in burns: a comprehensive review. Ann Burns Fire Disasters 26:147-153, 2013.

18. Moore EC, Padiglione AA, Wasiak J, et al. Candida in burns: risk factors and outcomes. J Burn Care Res 31:257-263, 2010.

19. Pruitt BA Jr, McManus AT. Opportunistic infections in severely burned patients. Am J Med 76:146-154, 1984.

20. Pruitt BA Jr. Host-opportunistic interactions in surgical infection. Arch Surg 121:13-22, 1986.

21. Lampe KF. Topical antiinfective agents: drugs used on skin and mucous membranes. In American Medical Association, ed. Drug Evaluations Annual, ed 7. Chicago: American Medical Association, 1991.

22. Moncrief JA. Topical antibacterial treatment of the burn patient. In Artz CP, Moncrief JA, Pruitt BA Jr, eds. Burns: A Team Approach. Philadelphia: WB Saunders, 1979.

23. Hansbrough JF, Achauer B, Dawson J, et al. Wound healing in partial thickness burns treated with collagenase ointment vs. silver sulfadiazine cream. J Burn Care Rehabil 16:241-247, 1995.

24. Greenhalgh DG. Topical antimicrobial agents for burn wounds. Clin Plast Surg 36:597-606, 2009.

25. LeVoyer T, Cioffi WG Jr, Pratt L, et al. Alterations in intestinal permeability after thermal injury. Arch Surg 127:26-29, 1992.
26. McCampbell B, Wasif N, Rabbitts A, et al. Diabetes and burns: retrospective cohort study. J Burn Care Rehabil 23:157-166, 2002.
27. Vanzant EL, Lopez CM, Ozrazgat-Baslanti T, et al. Persistent inflammation, immunosuppression, and catabolism syndrome after severe blunt trauma. J Trauma Acute Care Surg 76:21-29; discussion 29-30, 2014.
28. McManus AT, Mason AD Jr, McManus WF, et al. A decade of reduced gram-negative infections and mortality associated with improved isolation of burned patients. Arch Surg 129:1306-1309, 1994.
29. Pasteur L. Mémoire sur les corpuscles organisés qui existent dans l'atmosphère: examen de la doctrine des générations spontanées. Annales Sciences Naturelles 16:5-98, 1861.
30. Sheridan RL, Weber JM, Pasternack MS, et al. Antibiotic prophylaxis for group A streptococcal burn wound infection is not necessary. J Trauma 51:352-355, 2001.
31. Sheridan RL, Chang P. Acute burn procedures. Surg Clin North Am 94:755-764, 2014.
32. Singer AJ, McClain SA. Persistent wound infection delays epidermal maturation and increases scarring in thermal burns. Wound Repair Regen 10:372-377, 2002.
33. Keen A, Knoblock L, Edelman L, et al. Effective limitation of blood culture use in the burn unit. J Burn Care Rehabil 23:183-189, 2002.
34. Santucci SG, Gobara S, Santos CR, et al. Infections in a burn intensive care unit: experience of seven years. J Hosp Infect 53:6-13, 2003.
35. Appelgren P, Bjornhagen V, Bragderyd K, et al. A prospective study of infections in burn patients. Burns 28:39-46, 2002.
36. Sasaki TM, Welch GW, Herndon DN, et al. Burn wound manipulation induced bacteremia. J Trauma 19:46-48, 1979.
37. Estahbanati HK, Kashani PP, Ghanaatpisheh F. Frequency of Pseudomonas aeruginosa serotypes in burn wound infections and their resistance to antibiotics. Burns 28:340-348, 2002.
38. Signorini M, Grappolini S, Magliano E, et al. Updated evaluation of the activity of antibiotics in a burn centre. Burns 18:500-503, 1992.
39. Sheridan RL, Greenhalgh D. Special problems in burns. Surg Clin North Am 94:781-791, 2014.
40. Demling RH. Medical progress: burns. N Engl J Med 313:1389-1398, 1985.

6 Nutrition

KEY POINTS

- Burns cause a dramatic increase in metabolic rates.
- Burns result in large amounts of fluid losses.
- Protein requirements are increased, with a possible decrease in muscle mass.
- Enteral feedings are the best means of replacement.
- Some patients may require tube feeds even though they are taking nutrition orally.

Nutrition is of crucial importance in the care of burn patients. A burn patient is in a hypermetabolic state. This hypermetabolism is typically proportional to the extent of the injury and the accompanying responses, infections, and complications. A 50% increase in metabolism is expected in patients with multiple blunt injuries, central nervous system injuries, and major abdominal injuries, whereas a 100% increase in metabolism can be seen in patients with major burn injuries.[1,2]

It has been shown in burn patients that the cardiac index and oxygen consumption are proportional to the severity of the injury.[3] The upper limit of hypermetabolism seems to be 2 to 2.5 times the basal metabolic rate (BMR).[4] The rate of caloric expenditure and of protein catabolism are increased, resulting from the increased levels of catecholamines, glucagon, and glucocorticoids.[5] Moderate to severe stress can deplete nutrition, depress the immune system, decrease protein stores, diminish the inflammatory response, and interfere with wound healing.[1]

INJURY, METABOLIC RATE, AND STRESS FACTORS

The relative effects of injury on metabolism[6] are shown in Table 6-1.

A burn patient loses large amounts of heat through wounds, as previously discussed. This may be another factor contributing to hypermetabolism. In one study, burn patients' core and skin temperatures and metabolic rate remained elevated, even when the net heat loss was reduced by using increasing ambient temperatures.[7] Burn patients who were allowed to select their most comfortable ambient temperature consistently chose warmer temperatures than the control group. The findings were explained as a response to the injury increasing the central temperature set-point of the patient.[4]

The body's response to stress includes protein catabolism, with subsequent urinary nitrogen loss and muscle wasting. Each gram of

Table 6-1   Effects of Injury on Metabolism

Injury	Metabolic Activity (%)	Incidence in Stress Factor
Elective operation	0-5	1.00-1.05
Long-bone fracture	15-30	1.15-1.30
Multiple trauma	30-55	1.30-1.55
Multiple trauma and sepsis	50-75	1.50-1.75
10% Burn	25	1.25
20% Burn	50	1.50
30% Burn	70	1.70
40% Burn	85	1.85
50% Burn	100	2.00
75% Burn	100-110	2.00-2.10

nitrogen represents 6.25 g of protein (roughly 20 g of muscle). A patient undergoing starvation (e.g., an NPO patient) loses about 75 g of muscle protein per day (roughly 200 to 300 g of muscle tissue). A 60% increase in metabolism can translate into a loss of 250 g of muscle protein per day (roughly 750 to 1000 g of muscle mass). The protein is broken down through deamination of amino acids to provide carbon skeletons for glucose production (e.g., gluconeogenesis in the liver). This breakdown is, again, proportional to the severity of the stress.[8]

Skeletal muscle is the largest source of protein stores. These protein stores are utilized after burn injury. In a study in which amino acid release from the legs of patients with major burns was measured, the release of amino acid nitrogen increased fivefold.[9] Branched-chain amino acids (BCAAs) are leucine, isoleucine, and valine. They are oxidized primarily in muscle, and the breakdown of muscle releases these amino acids in large amounts. They are also known to stimulate the secretion of insulin.[10] Providing high levels of BCAAs in nutritional support may decrease muscle breakdown; however, more studies are needed before a definitive statement can be made.[1,11]

Glutamine is a unique amino acid; it is sometimes referred to as a *conditionally essential amino acid.* The requirements of glutamine can be significantly increased in a stressed patient. Glutamine represents one third of the nitrogen derived through catabolic metabolism of amino acids, and it has many uses.[10] This is especially true for the rapidly dividing cells of the GI tract. Glutamine-enriched parenteral nutrition nourishes the enterocytes, protects against atrophy of the intestinal mucosa, and improves nitrogen retention.[12] Maintenance of intestinal integrity may decrease translocation of bacteria and cytokines across the GI barrier, thus decreasing the incidence of sepsis.[13-15] Provision of glutamine may also be important for maintenance of a patient's immunologic responses.[16] Levels of glutamine are decreased in stress states, and it needs to be a part of the nutritional plan.[10,17,18]

Other pharmacologic interventions have been studied in an effort to prevent muscle breakdown during recovery from burns (e.g., testosterone, oxandrolone, human recombinant growth hormone, insulin, metformin, and propranolol).[19]

Hyperglycemia is noted after injury and is primarily caused by increased glucose production. The extra glucose comes from the synthesis from amino acids and glucose recycled from lactate. The fasting glucose and serum insulin concentrations are elevated. The elevations are not proportionate, and the normal insulin-glucose relationship and insulin resistance may be disturbed.[4,20]

Lipolysis is also increased in burn patients, by several mechanisms—the firing of sympathetic nerves releases adipose stores and the increased levels of cortisol, catecholamines, and glucagon. This lipolysis is not suppressed by increased glucose levels. However, the availability of lipid is decreased as the circulation to the adipose tissue is impaired, decreasing free fatty acid (FFA) mobilization. The body may not be able to utilize triglycerides and FFAs, because the activity of lipoprotein lipase may decrease.[21] Hormone-sensitive lipase (the lipase found in cells that actively breaks down triglycerides in adipose sites) may also be decreased.

These metabolic findings are coordinated to elicit a response beneficial to the patient. Multiple organ systems work together to attempt to supply injured tissue with the oxygen and metabolites needed for healing. They are regulated by neuroendocrine pathways through a variety of agents (cortisol, glucagon, thyroid hormones, catecholamines, insulin, growth hormone, and cytokines).[20,22]

NUTRITIONAL SUPPORT

Early and adequate nutritional support will minimize lean body mass catabolism, improve immune function, and protect protein synthesis. Enteral feedings are safer and less expensive than parenteral feedings and should be used whenever possible.[23] Enteral feedings also protect the integrity of the bowel lumen[21]; this will decrease bacterial and toxin translocation into the peritoneal space and bloodstream.[13] Limiting translocation will decrease cytokine responses and involvement of the lungs (as the peritoneal lymph channels move lymph toward the diaphragm). The risk of infection is reduced in burn patients who are supported by earliest possible enteral nutrition.[24] In our institution, enteral feedings are started as soon as feasible.[25-27] When the patient is admitted, an NGT is used to empty the stomach, and then 100 ml of a high-glutamine feeding formula is given in the stomach. The tube is clamped for 30 to 45 minutes. The NGT is then placed to suction, and enteral feedings are begun if the gastric residuals are less than 100 ml/hr and active bowel sounds are present.[28] Postpyloric tubes are usually placed after the first day if the patient is tolerating tube feeds. PEG tubes are usually placed at the time of the tracheotomy, on approximately day 10 to 14 after the injury. If the patient is not tolerating stomach feedings after the PEG, it can be changed to a percutaneous jejunostomy tube after approximately 1 week, when a good tract is formed. Our success rate is approximately 90% using an endoscope. The postpyloric port is used for feeding, and the stomach can be decompressed with the gastric port. If a patient suddenly stops tolerating feedings and has high residuals, it may be an early sign that sepsis is starting.

Caloric and Protein Needs

Determining the patient's energy needs and BMR is necessary for the initiation of nutritional support. This is an estimate, a starting point. Adjustments will be made after evaluation of nutritional parameters. Many formulas can be used to estimate the basal energy expenditure (BEE):

- **Method 1**   A common and accurate formula to estimate the basal energy expenditure is the Harris-Benedict equation[29]:

Male = 66.5 × (13.7 × Weight in kg) + (5 × Height in cm) − (6.8 × Age)
Female = 65.5 + (9.6 × Weight in kg) + (1.7 × Height in cm) − (4.7 × Age)

The patient's normal preinjury weight is used for the calculation. Patients will gain a significant amount of weight with edema from the fluid resuscitation.

A stress factor needs to be added to the BEE to account for the increased metabolic needs of the patient. Burns greater than 20% of the body surface area (BSA) cause severe stress, and the BMR should be multiplied by a factor of 2. Burns less than 20% have a moderate stress level, and the BMR should be multiplied by a factor of 1.6.

- **Method 2** An alternative method can be used to obtain a starting point. The caloric requirement can be estimated at 40 to 50 kcal/kg for severe stress. For moderate stress, the estimated need is 35 to 40 kcal/kg.
- **Method 3** The basal energy expenditure is estimated to be 25 kcal/kg; this is multiplied by the stress factor used in method 1 (i.e., 1.6 for moderate stress, 2.0 for high stress).
- **Method 4** Another method uses the Curreri formula:

$$\text{Amount of calories needed} = (25 \text{ kcal} \times \text{kg}) + (40 \text{ kcal} \times \% \text{ total burned surface area [TBSA]})$$

The energy expenditure can be accurately calculated with a variety of other methods (e.g., the Fick principle and Weir equation, the metabolic cart, and differential oximetry), but in clinical application, only a starting point is needed. The patient's nutritional status is monitored weekly (using prealbumin and transferrin levels). Some institutions now have handheld metabolic cart units. The data at a particular institution can be evaluated and adjustments made.[30-32]

Fat is a dense source of calories. Usually, it is desirable for 30% of calories to come from fat. Special considerations in pulmonary disease may require an increase of fats to 60% of the daily requirement to lower the respiratory quotient (CO_2/O_2) and decrease CO_2 production (Table 6-2). In patients with respiratory difficulty, it may be advisable to give more calories as fat to decrease the amount of CO_2

Table 6-2 Respiratory Quotient

Carbohydrates	1.0
Protein	0.8
Lipids	0.7

Table 6-3 Protein Needs Vary With Stress Levels

No stress	1 g/kg/day
Moderate stress	1.5-2.2 g/kg/day
High stress	2.2-3.2 g/kg/day

produced. This may improve the respiratory status, and the patient may wean more easily from the ventilator. The patient should receive at least 1000 kcal/wk as fat to prevent essential fatty acid deficiency.

The normal respiratory quotient is 0.8 in an average adult diet, consisting of 70% carbohydrate calories and 30% fat calories. After the caloric needs are estimated, the protein needs are calculated. Protein calories "do not count" toward the caloric needs of the patient. Normal protein intake is 1 g/kg/day. Moderately stressed patients need 1.5 to 2.2 g of protein/kg/day. Patients with severe stress, such as a burn injury, require 2.2 to 3.2 g of protein/kg/day (Table 6-3).

The ratio of calories to grams of nitrogen in a healthy, non-stressed individual is 300:1. In the hospital, the ratio usually used is 150:1 (because the patients are usually under stress). The quotient is then multiplied by 6.25 (6.25 g of protein per gram of nitrogen). This gives the grams of protein needed. The more stressed the patient, the lower the calorie/nitrogen ratio (i.e., 100:1 for very stressed patients).

[Calories/150] × 6.25 = Grams of protein needed (for moderate stress)

ASSESSMENT OF PROTEIN NUTRITIONAL STATUS

The nitrogen balance (how much protein a patient needs) can be obtained from a 24-hour urinary urea nitrogen (UUN) measurement. The usual formula is:

$$\text{Total nitrogen loss (TNL)} = \text{UUN} + 4 \text{ g}$$

6.25 g of protein is required to receive 1 g of biologically available nitrogen. Therefore:

$$\text{Protein needs} = \text{TNL} \times 6.25$$

The goal of therapy is a positive nitrogen balance of 2 to 4 g of nitrogen (15 to 30 g of protein) per day.[30] For example, for protein intake:

How many grams of protein given/6.25 = Grams of nitrogen given
Grams of nitrogen given − (UUN + 4) = Nitrogen balance (+ or −)

Again, the number should be positive.

Specifically, in a burn patient, the TNL (Table 6-4) can be estimated as follows:

$$\text{TNL} = 2 + \text{24-hr UUN} + \text{Wound nitrogen loss}$$

This is an estimate of the initial needs of the patient. The patient's nutritional status requires monitoring (usually once a week), and adjustments can be made accordingly. The UUN is an accurate estimate of the total urinary nitrogen in a burn-injured patient.[33]

Table 6-4 Total Nitrogen Loss

Total Burned Surface Area (%)	Nitrogen/kg/day Wound Loss
<10	0.02 g nitrogen/kg/day wound loss
10-30	0.05 g nitrogen/kg/day wound loss
>30	0.12 g nitrogen/kg/day wound loss

Fluids

The Parkland formula is used as a starting point for fluid resuscitation.

Initial fluid replacement with lactated Ringer's solution is computed for the first 24 hours of treatment. The equation, as mentioned before, is:

$$4 \text{ ml LR} \times \text{Body weight in kg} \times \%\text{TBSA}$$

Calculation of fluid resuscitation begins from the time of injury, not when the patient arrives in the emergency department. The first half of this volume is given within 8 hours of the burn (even if transfer of the patient to a medical center is delayed). The second half is given over the next 16 hours.

During the fourth 8-hour postburn period, salt-poor albumin (SPA) is infused, using the equation $(0.1 \times \text{kg} \times \%\text{TBSA})$. Some burn units will administer free water in addition to the maintenance fluids for patients with more than 25% TBSA. Our unit will be mindful of the evaporative losses until the wound is covered. We typically add free water if the patient becomes hypernatremic. The calculation for water evaporation is:

$$\%\text{TBSA} + (25 \times \text{body surface area [BSA] in m}^2) =$$
$$\text{Number of milliliters of evaporative water loss/hr}$$

Remember that BSA should not be confused with TBSA. BSA is calculated as follows:

$$[87 (H + W) - 2600] \div 10{,}000 = \text{Surface in m}^2$$

where H = Height in cm; W = weight in kg. This amount is replaced as free water. Evaluation of serum Na will give an indication of adequate replacement. The optimal level of Na to be maintained is 135 to 137 mg/dl. As the slope of the curve of Na levels changes, trends can be determined and corrected before increased losses are present. After the first 24-hour resuscitation period, the maintenance fluid is ½ NS. Maintenance fluids are based on the patient (see BSA

Table 6-5   Administration Rate of Maintenance Fluids

First 10 kg	100 ml/kg
Second 10 kg	50 ml/kg
Every kg above 20 kg	20 ml/kg

calculation in Chapter 3), with close monitoring of the I&O. The rate is calculated for 24 hours using the guideline shown in Table 6-5.

For example, a 70 kg patient's calculation is 100×10 (for the first 10 kg) + 50×10 (for the second 10 kg) + 20×50 (for the 50 kg not covered yet): $1000 + 500 + 1000 = 2500$ ml/24 hr. The total is 104 ml/hr. This is an estimate and can be rounded up to a more workable number (i.e., 105 ml/hr).

Close observation is needed during fluid resuscitation, because too much fluid early can result in bowel edema and secondary abdominal compartment syndrome.[34-36]

Electrolytes

The amount of sodium required ranges from 60 to 200 mEq/day. Less is required in patients with cardiac and renal failure. The amount of potassium needed is 50 to 160 mEq/day. Patients will need more if they are stressed, on NGT suction, with a hyperinsulin state, or have a metabolic alkalosis. Chloride requirements are 100 to 200 mEq/day, more with gastric loss. Calcium requirements range from 4 to 30 mEq. Magnesium requirements are 8 to 24 mEq. Phosphate requirements are 30 to 100 mEq. In the burn unit, the standard solution is ½ NS + 20 mEq KCl. This can be adjusted, and repletion of electrolytes can be given as guided by laboratory analysis.

Vitamins

A multivitamin and minerals are given, as described in Chapter 3. Repletion of other vitamins and minerals should be clinically based.[37]

Trace Elements

Trace elements are essential enzymatic cofactors in a variety of metabolic reactions. Zinc, manganese, copper, and chromium are added to parenteral solutions daily, along with the vitamins.

Zinc and iron levels are decreased by acute-phase reactants. The benefits of adding zinc are currently under much study. Bacteremia also tends to decrease the iron level. It is proposed that the bacteria need this element for biochemical reactions. Ongoing studies are evaluating withholding of iron in septic patients. A study of patients with significant burns noted a decrease in the duration of hospitalization in the increased trace mineral intake group.[38]

Antioxidants

Antioxidants may prevent the damage caused by free radicals produced in the stress states. Copper and selenium are known to be involved in immune responses, oxidative defense mechanisms, and tissue repair.[39] Important nutrients and their activity are listed in Table 6-6.

ENTERAL VERSUS PARENTERAL FEEDINGS

Most physicians will agree that if a patient's gastrointestinal tract can be used, then it should be used. This will help to maintain the benefits of nutritional support, including maintenance of the integrity of the gut (thus preventing bacterial translocation). It will also prevent the possible complications associated with total parenteral nutrition (TPN). If a patient's GI tract cannot be accessed (guideline of 7 days), or if using the enteral route is contraindicated, then nutritional support with a parenteral route is warranted[14,28,40,41] (Table 6-7).

Many enteral feeding formulas are commercially available. Dietitians can be quite valuable in selecting the proper formulation for each patient. In our burn unit, feedings are started immediately if possible. We determine the patient's BEE + stress factor. The goal feeding is then calculated. The strength and rate of the feedings are increased per the protocol described next (if tolerated by the patient).

EXAMPLE: NPO if burn >30%:

> Enteral feedings, TraumaCal or similar:
>
> > Target feedings of 25 kcal/kg/day × 2.0 (stress factor)
>
> Tube feedings:
>
> > ½ strength @ 25 ml/hr × 4 hr, then
> >
> > ¾ strength @ 25 ml/hr × 4 hr, then
> >
> > Full strength @ 25 ml/hr × 4 hr, then
> >
> > Increase 15 ml/q4h to goal
>
> Check residuals q4h. Hold if >150 ml. If <150 ml, feed the aspirate back to the patient.

Table 6-6 Vitamins and Minerals and Their Properties

Nutrient	Activity
Vitamin C	Direct cytosolic antioxidant
Vitamin E	Direct antioxidant with action primarily at the cell membrane
Beta carotene	Antioxidant properties, particularly at the membrane lipid
Zinc	Constituent of superoxide dismutase in cytosol
Manganese	Constituent of superoxide dismutase in mitochondria
Copper	Constituent of superoxide dismutase, and of the scavenger ceruloplasmin
Iron	Constituent of catalase
Selenium	Constituent of glutathione peroxidase
Glutamine	Substrate for endogenous glutathione

From Youn YK, LaLonde C, Demling R. Use of antioxidant therapy in shock and trauma. Circ Shock 35:245-249, 1991.

Table 6-7 Complications of Parenteral Feedings

Mechanical	Air or catheter embolism, pneumothorax, hemothorax, hydrothorax, arterial laceration, catheter tip malposition, venous thrombosis
Infectious	Catheter-related sepsis
Acute metabolic	Hyperglycemia, hypoglycemia, serum electrolyte abnormalities, fluid overload, hyperlipidemia
Prolonged use	Metabolic bone disease, intestinal mucosal atrophy, bacterial overgrowth, bacterial translocation, deterioration of liver function, alteration in bile composition

Table 6-8   Enteral Feeding Formulas

	Product	Standard formulas		Specialty formulas: Disease specific				
		Jevity	TwoCal HN	Nepro	Suplena	Pulmocare	NutriHep	Glucerna
1	Classification	Standard isotonic with fiber	2 Kcal/ml High calorie High protein	High calorie High protein Low electrolytes	High calorie Low protein Low electrolytes	Low carbohydrate	High branch chain amino acids (AA) Low aromatic AA	High fat Low CHO
2	Tube, oral, or both	Both	Both			Both	Both	Both
3	Calories/ml	1.06	2.0	2.0	2.0	1.5	1.5	1.0
4	Osmolality	310	690	635	600	475	690	355
5	Protein (g/ml)	0.044	0.084	0.070	0.030	0.063	0.040	0.042
6	Fat (g/ml)	0.035	0.091	0.096	0.095	0.093	0.021	0.054
7	Carbohydrate (g/ml)	0.152	0.217	0.215	0.255	0.106	0.290	0.096
8	Nonprotein Cal:N ratio	125:1	125:1	179:1	393:1	125:1	209:1	125:1
9	Protein source	Sodium & calcium caseinates	Sodium & calcium caseinates	Calcium, sodium, & magnesium caseinates	Sodium & calcium caseinates	Sodium & calcium caseinates	L-Amino acids Whey protein (50% BCCA)	Sodium & calcium caseinates
10	Fat source	High-oleic safflower oil (50%) Canola oil (30%) MCT oil (20%)	Corn oil MCT oil	High-oleic safflower oil (90%) Soy oil (10%)	High-oleic safflower oil (90%) Soy oil (10%)	Canola oil MCT oil Corn oil High-oleic safflower oil	MCT oil (66%) Canola oil Soy lecithin Corn oil	High-oleic safflower oil Canola oil Soy lecithin
11	Carbohydrate source	Hydrolyzed corn-starch, soy poly-saccharide	Maltodextrin, sucrose	Hydrolyzed cornstarch	Hydrolyzed cornstarch, sucrose, oat fiber, soy fiber	Sucrose, maltodextrin	Maltodextrin, modified cornstarch	Maltodextrin, soy fiber, fructose
12	Sodium (mg/ml)	0.930	1.456	0.829	0.783	1.310	0.320	0.930
13	Potassium (mg/ml)	1.570	2.456	1.057	1.116	1.730	1.360	1.570
14	Magnesium (mg/ml)	0.304	0.421	0.211	0.211	0.423	0.178	0.282
15	Phosphorus (mg/ml)	0.758	1.052	0.686	0.728	1.056	0.445	0.704
16	Calcium (mg/ml)	0.904	1.052	1.373	1.385	1.056	0.445	0.704
17	% Free water	84%	71%	70%	71%	79%	76%	87%
18	Milliliters needed to meet RDAs	1321	947	960 ml needed to meet RDAs, except Phos, Mg, vitamins A & D, which are limited in renal diets	947	947	1000	1422
19	Comments	Lactose free 14.4 g fiber/L.	Concentrated for fluid restricted patients Lactose free Gluten free	Tailored for patients with renal failure who receive dialysis	Tailored for patients with renal failure, pre-dialysis Gluten free Lactose free Low residue	Low CHO to reduce CO₂ production in respiratory failure Lactose free Gluten free	Tailored for chronic liver disease BCAA aromatic & methionine	Tailored for unstable diabetics whose blood sugars are out of control Not recommended for long-term use
20	Expense	$	$	$$	$	$	$$$$$	$$
21	Supplier	Ross	Ross	Ross	Ross	Ross	Nestle	Ross

#	Critical care formulas			Oral supplements per serving size					Tube feeding/Oral modifiers	
	Peptamen	Perative	Crucial	Ensure Plus	Resource	Ensure pudding	Health shakes	Sugar free health shakes	MCT oil	ProMod
1	Semi-elemental Isotonic	Semi-elemental High protein	Semi-elemental High calorie High protein	8 oz	8 oz clear liquid	5 oz	6 oz	6 oz	15 ml/Tbsp	6.6 g protein/scoop
2	Tube	Tube	Tube	Oral	Oral	Oral	Oral	Oral	Both	Both
3	1.0	1.3	1.5	355	180/8 oz	250/5 oz	280/6 oz	290/6 oz	7.75/ml	28 Kcal/scoop
4	270	385	490	450	700	700	—	—		
5	0.04	0.067	0.094	13.2	8.8 g/8 oz	7 g/5 oz	9 g/6 oz	12 g/6 oz	14 g/Tbsp	5 g/scoop
6	0.039	0.038	0.068	12.7	0 g/8 oz	10 g/5 oz	6 g/6 oz	9 g/6 oz	—	—
7	127	0.177	0.135	48	36 g/8 oz	34 g/5 oz	48 g/6 oz	40 g/6 oz	—	—
8	131:1	97:1	67:1	150:1	105:1	230:1	—	—	—	—
9	Protein hydrolysate & peptides	Hydrolyzed sodium & caseinates & lactalbumin hydrolysates L-Arginine	Enzymatically hydrolyzed casein L-Arginine	Sodium & calcium caseinates soy protein isolate	Whey protein concentrate	Nonfat milk	Skim & nonfat dry milk	Skim milk, milk protein concentrate	—	Whey protein concentrate, soy lecithin
10	MCT oil (70%) Sunflower oil (30%)	Canola oil (40%) MCT oil (40%) Corn oil (20%)	MCT oil (50%) Marine oil (25%) Soy oil (25%)	Corn oil (100%)	No fat	Partially hydrogenated soybean oil	Corn oil	Corn oil	Medium chain triglycerides (100%)	—
11	Maltodextrin, cornstarch	Maltodextrin, cornstarch	Maltodextrin, cornstarch	Maltodextrin, sucrose	Sucrose, hydrolyzed cornstarch	Lactose, sucrose, modified food starch	—	—	—	—
12	0.500	1.040	1.170	280/8 oz	55/8 oz	239.2/5 oz	140/6 oz	240/6 oz	—	—
13	1.250	1.730	1.870	430/8 oz	15/8 oz	237/5 oz	400/6 oz	380/6 oz	—	—
14	0.400	0.347	0.400	100/8 oz	50/8 oz	68/5 oz	—	—	—	—
15	0.700	0.867	1.000	250/8 oz	160/8 oz	200/5 oz	—	—	—	—
16	0.800	0.867	1.000	250/8 oz	135/8 oz	200/5 oz	—	—	—	—
17	85%	79%	77%	182/8 oz	Approx 200 cc/8 oz	—	—	—	—	—
18	1500	1155	1000	1420	1900	Not applicable	—	—	—	—
19	For impaired GI function (i.e., short bowel syndrome, IBD, malabsorption, pancreatic insufficiency, chronic diarrhea, & radiation)	Lactose free L-Arginine & beta-carotene enriched	Lactose free Glutamin & arginine enriched	Lactose free Vanilla, chocolate, & strawberry	Clear liquid supplement Fat free Very low K+ & Na+ Low residue Lactose free	Gluten free Used for patients with impaired ability to swallow or fluid restriction NOT lactose free	House oral supplement	Diabetic house oral supplement	Supplemental MCT easily digested & absorbed	Supplemental high quality protein from whey Very low lactose
20 / 21	$$$$$ Nestle	$$$ Ross	$$$$$ Nestle	$ Ross	$ Sandoz	$ Ross	$ Sandoz	$ Sandoz	$$	$$ Ross

Table 6-8 presents a listing of the enteral feedings available. Note the location of the feeding catheter. In feedings to the stomach, tonicity is increased first, then volume is increased. With feedings to the small bowel, volume is increased first, then tonicity is increased (to prevent diarrhea). The patient's nutritional status is assessed regularly. The UUN is used for computing the nitrogen balance and guides protein administration. Transferrin, prealbumin, and albumin are used to evaluate general nutritional therapy.

REFERENCES

1. Van Way CW III. Nutritional support in the injured patient. Surg Clin North Am 71:537-548, 1991.
2. Chan MM, Chan GM. Nutritional therapy for burns in children and adults. Nutrition 25:261-269, 2009.
3. Wilmore DW, Aulich LH, Mason AD, et al. Influence of the burn wound on local and systemic responses to injury. Ann Surg 186:444-458, 1977.
4. Bessey PQ. Parenteral nutrition and trauma. In Rombeau JL, Rolandelli RH, eds. Clinical Nutrition: Parenteral Nutrition, ed 3. Philadelphia: WB Saunders, 2001.
5. Clifton GL, Robertson CS, Grossman RG, et al. The metabolic response to severe head injury. J Neurosurg 60:687-696, 1984.
6. Wilmore DW, ed. The Metabolic Management of the Critically Ill. New York: Plenum, 1977.
7. Wilmore DW, Mason AD Jr, Johnson DW, et al. Effect of ambient temperature on heat production and heat loss in burn patients. J Appl Physiol 38:593-597, 1975.
8. Goodwin C. Metabolism and nutrition in the thermally injured patient. Crit Care Clin 1:97-117, 1985.
9. Aulick LH, Wilmore DW. Increased peripheral amino acid release following burn injury. Surgery 85:560-565, 1979.
10. Wilmore DW. Catabolic illness. Strategies for enhancing recovery. N Engl J Med 325:695-702, 1991.
11. Wandrag L, Brett SJ, Frost G, et al. Impact of supplementation with amino acids or their metabolites on muscle wasting in patients with critical illness or other muscle wasting illness: a systematic review. J Hum Nutr Diet 28:313-330, 2015.
12. O'Dwyer ST, Smith RJ, Hwang TL, et al. Maintenance of small bowel mucosa with glutamine-enriched parenteral nutrition. JPEN J Parenteral Enter Nutr 13:579-585, 1989.

13. Maejima K, Deitch E, Berg RD. Bacterial translocation from the gastrointestinal tracts of rats receiving thermal injury. Infect Immun 43:86-102, 1984.

14. LeVoyer T, Cioffi WG Jr, Pratt L, et al. Alterations in intestinal permeability after thermal injury. Arch Surg 127:26-29, 1992.

15. Wischmeyer PE, Lynch J, Liedel J, et al. Glutamine administration reduces gram-negative bacteremia in severely burned patients: a prospective, randomized, double-blind trial versus isonitrogenous control. Crit Care Med 29:2075-2080, 2001.

16. Lacey JM, Wilmore DW. Is glutamine a conditionally essential amino acid? Nutr Rev 48:297-309, 1990.

17. Souba WW, Klimberg VS, Plumley DA, et al. The role of glutamine in maintaining a healthy gut and supporting the metabolic response to injury and infection. J Surg Res 48:383-391, 1990.

18. Lin JJ, Chung XJ, Yang CY, et al. A meta-analysis of trials using the intention to treat principle for glutamine supplementation in critically ill patients with burn. Burns 39:565-570, 2013.

19. Diaz EC, Herndon DN, Porter C, et al. Effects of pharmacological interventions on muscle protein synthesis and breakdown in recovery from burns. Burns 41:649-657, 2015.

20. Thomas SJ, Morimoto K, Herndon DN, et al. The effect of prolonged euglycemic hyperinsulinemia on lean body mass after severe burn. Surgery 132:341-347, 2002.

21. Frankel WL, Evans NJ, Rombeau JL. Scientific rationale and clinical application of parenteral nutrition in critically ill patients. In Rombeau JL, Rolandelli RH, eds. Clinical Nutrition: Parenteral Nutrition, ed 3. Philadelphia: WB Saunders, 2001.

22. Williams GJ, Herndon DN. Modulating the hypermetabolic response to burn injuries. J Wound Care 11:87-89, 2002.

23. Mandell SP, Gibran NS. Early enteral nutrition for burn injury. Adv Wound Care (New Rochelle) 3:64-70, 2014.

24. Lu G, Huang J, Yu J, et al. Influence of early post-burn enteral nutrition on clinical outcomes of patients with extensive burns. J Clin Biochem Nutr 48:222-225, 2011.

25. Holt B, Graves C, Faraklas I, et al. Compliance with nutrition support guidelines in acutely burned patients. Burns 38:645-649, 2012.

26. Hall KL, Shahrokhi S, Jeschke MG. Enteral nutrition support in burn care: a review of current recommendations as instituted in the Ross Tilley Burn Centre. Nutrients 4:1554-1165, 2012.

27. Rousseau AF, Losser MR, Ichai C, et al. ESPEN endorsed recommendations: nutritional therapy in major burns. Clin Nutr 32:497-502, 2013.

28. McClave SA, Marsano LS, Lukan JK. Enteral access for nutritional support: rationale for utilization. J Clin Gastroenterol 35:209-213, 2002.

29. Harris J, Benedict F. A biometric study of basal metabolism in man. Publ No. 279, Carnegie Institute of Washington. Philadelphia: JB Lippincott, 1919, as cited in American Dietetic Association Manual of Clinical Dietetics, Chicago, 1988.

30. Long CL, Schaffel N, Geiger JW, et al. Metabolic response to injury and illness: estimation of energy and protein needs from indirect calorimetry and nitrogen balance. JPEN J Parenteral Enter Nutr 3:452-457, 1979.

31. Williamson J. Actual burn nutrition care practices: a national survey (Part II). J Burn Care Rehab 10:185-194, 1989.

32. Dickerson RN, Gervasio JM, Riley ML, et al. Accuracy of predictive methods to estimate resting energy expenditure of thermally-injured patients. JPEN J Parenteral Enter Nutr 26:17-29, 2002.

33. Milner EA, Cioffi WG Jr, Mason AD Jr, et al. Accuracy of urinary urea nitrogen for predicting total urinary nitrogen in thermally injured patients. JPEN J Parenteral Enter Nutr 17:414-426, 1993.

34. McBeth PB, Sass K, Nickerson D, et al. A necessary evil? Intra-abdominal hypertension complicating burn patient resuscitation. J Trauma Manag Outcomes 8:12, 2014.

35. Strang SG, Van Lieshout EM, Breederveld RS, et al. A systematic review on intra-abdominal pressure in severely burned patients. Burns 40:9-16, 2014.

36. Cancio LC. Initial assessment and fluid resuscitation of burn patients. Surg Clin North Am 94:741-754, 2014.

37. Van Way CW III. Vitamin and mineral deficiency. Handbook Surg Nutr 58:31-42, 1992.

38. Berger MM, Cavadini C, Chiolero R, et al. Influence of large intakes of trace elements on recovery after major burns. Nutrition 10:327-334, 1994.

39. Youn YK, LaLonde C, Demling R. Use of antioxidant therapy in shock and trauma. Circ Shock 35:245-249, 1991.

40. American Society for Parenteral and Enteral Nutrition. Guidelines for the use of parenteral and enteral nutrition in adult and pediatric patients. JPEN J Parenteral Enter Nutr 17(4 Suppl):1SA-52SA, 1993.

41. Kreis BE, Middelkoop E, Vloemans AF, et al. The use of a PEG tube in a burn centre. Burns 28:191-197, 2002.

7 Inhalation Injury

KEY POINTS

- Inhalation injury significantly affects burn patients.
- Clinical issues can appear late; therefore physicians should maintain a high index of suspicion.
- Carbon monoxide and toxins should be suspected.
- Aggressive pulmonary toilet may be needed.
- The patient's arterial blood gas (ABG) should be obtained after every ventilator adjustment.

Inhalation injury is common, especially in patients with severe burns. It is an indicator of a poor prognosis. Mortality rates with inhalation injury usually are reported to be between 30% and 40%, and the mortality rate without inhalation injury is reported to be between 4% and 7%.[1-3] The incidence is lower in children, who have a higher percentage of scald injury than adults. Inhalation injury can be diagnosed by history and physical examination, laboratory studies, chest radiographs, and fiberscopic examination. The pulmonary injury is usually proportional to the depth and size of the cutaneous burn.[4-6]

Although mortality from smoke inhalation alone is low (0% to 11% of patients), smoke inhalation in combination with cutaneous burns is fatal in 30% to 90% of patients. Reports have indicated that the presence of inhalation injury increases burn mortality by 20% and that inhalation injury predisposes to pneumonia. Pneumonia has been shown to independently increase burn mortality by 40%. The combination of inhalation injury and pneumonia increases mortality by 60%. Children and the elderly are especially prone to pneumonia because of their limited physiologic reserve. A well-organized, protocol-driven approach to respiratory care of inhalation injury is imperative for improving care and decreasing morbidity and mortality from inhalation injury.[7,8]

Inhalational injuries can be acute, as in upper airway injury from heat damage, small airway damage from heat and particulate matter, and carbon monoxide poisoning. Toxins play a significant role, especially in victims of house fires, because many synthetic fabrics and home furnishings produce toxins when heated.[9]

Oxygen consumed during combustion decreases the ambient oxygen content in the air. This situation may lead to hypoxia in a person exposed to such an atmosphere for any length of time. Carbon monoxide poisoning, which is also common in structural fires, can be diagnosed by unconsciousness, a change in mental status, and the results of laboratory studies (increased carboxyhemoglobin, low oxygen saturation in relation to PaO_2, and unexplained acidosis).

Carbon monoxide poisoning can also result in the need for prolonged intubation. The classic cherry-red skin coloration associated with carbon monoxide poisoning is difficult to detect in burn patients. Symptoms will increase with increasing carboxyhemoglobin levels[9-11] (Table 7-1).

Table 7-1 The Increase in Symptoms Associated With Increasing Carboxyhemoglobin Levels

Carboxyhemoglobin Level (%)	Symptoms
0-10	Normal
10-20	Slight headache, confusion, dilation of cutaneous blood vessels
20-30	Headache, throbbing in the temples
30-40	Disorientation, fatigue, nausea, vomiting, visual disturbances
40-60	Combativeness, hallucinations, shock state, coma, intermittent convulsions, Cheyne-Stokes respirations
>60	Mortality rate of 50%
60-70	Coma, intermittent convulsions, depressed cardiac and respiratory function
70-80	Weak pulse, slow respirations, death within hours
80-90	Death in less than 1 hour
90-100	Death within minutes

Treatment modalities include 100% oxygen given by face mask. Treatment with 100% oxygen for 40 minutes will decrease a patient's carbon monoxide level by half.

Upper respiratory injury usually can be diagnosed based on a history of fire in an enclosed space, burns of the face, singed nasal hair, inflamed pharyngeal mucosa, carbonaceous sputum, and evidence of edematous glottis (e.g., hoarseness). Any two of these clinical signs should prompt high suspicion of an inhalation injury. Worsening hoarseness, stridor, an increased respiratory rate, and the inability to handle secretions indicate a worsening injury that will require intubation. Bronchoscopy is warranted in patients with hoarseness or increasing hoarseness. Patients with stridor should be intubated immediately.

Signs of lower airway damage usually present within 24 hours of the injury. Breath sounds characteristically are wheezing. Progressive hypoxemia may also develop. Intubation should be considered after hypoxemia or edema is confirmed.

Oxygenation by intubation is a mainstay of treatment of a pulmonary injury. For patients who are awake and alert, nasotracheal intubation is preferred over orotracheal intubation and can be accomplished even if a patient's teeth are clenched. The oral route of intubation is less stable, but the danger of sinusitis is avoided. The endotracheal tube is securely tied to ensure that it will not dislocate. Tape will not adhere to burned skin. Umbilical tape should be used and tied to the endotracheal tube and around the back of the head.

One treatment for inhalation injury is inhaled nitrous oxide. This treatment is used to reduce a ventilation/perfusion (V/Q) mismatch by dilating the pulmonary vessels perfusing ventilated alveoli. Nitrous oxide inhalation therapy does not work well in bacteremic patients. Anecdotal success has been reported in burn patients.

Another treatment modality is inhaled nebulized heparin mixed with albuterol. This has shown some success in decreasing airway casts.[12,13]

Byrd ventilators have significantly improved treatment. These combine oscillatory or high-frequency (500 to 800 breaths/min) treatment with pressure-controlled breaths. The use of these ventilators has led to a decrease in inspiratory pressures and decreased barotraumas with sufficient oxygenation. The oscillatory breaths also provide internal chest physical therapy, mobilizing and decreasing particulate matter in the airway. Studies from the Institute of Surgical Research have shown decreased morbidity and mortality using this ventilator system.[14] In our burn unit, the use of these ventilators has decreased the rate of pneumonia.

A circumferential chest burn can cause respiratory embarrassment by restricting chest movement as a result of edema. The swelling is restricted by the eschar, which is nonelastic and restricts chest excursion and breathing. An escharotomy may be necessary using the techniques described in Chapter 3.

PATHOPHYSIOLOGY

Damage to the upper airway is manifested by edema, erythema, and ulceration. Edema results from direct microvascular injury, oxygen free radicals, and inflammatory mediators. Pulmonary edema formation usually begins immediately, or may be delayed up to 24 hours. The administration of crystalloid solution in and of itself does not seem to be a contributing factor in lung edema.[15] The tongue, arytenoids, and epiglottis may swell, narrowing or closing the airway. The presence of the cartilaginous rings surrounding the glottis displaces swelling inward and narrows the airway. Edema usually resolves in 4 to 5 days. Decreases in upper airway edema can be estimated by evaluating the eyelids. When the edema of the eyelids has subsided, in general, the edema of the airway has also subsided and extubation should be considered.[16,17]

In contrast to the upper airway, the lower airways sustain less injury from dry heat. The upper airway can cool the warm air effectively. The vocal cords close at 150° C (302° F) and tend to serve as a protective measure. Steam has 4000 times the carrying capacity of dry air and can cause thermal injury. Smoke can carry superheated particles or soot into the lower airway system. These particles cause direct thermal injury to the mucosa by contact. Small airway occlusion secondary to sloughed endobronchial debris and the loss of the ciliary clearance mechanism can result in a high rate of pneumonia (20% to 50%).[4] Various chemical agents (e.g., aldehydes, acrolein, and acids) are released through burning. This is especially true of plastics, which can produce cyanide. Cyanide interferes with oxidative phosphorylation at the cellular level and causes metabolic acidosis. Specific treatment with sodium thiosulfate is not usually required in patients who have received adequate resuscitation and ventilation therapy.[18] Cyanide toxicity should only be treated if the pH remains low (7.0).

Constriction and obstruction of the airway cause vasoconstriction and hypoxia. Neutrophils are entrapped in the parenchyma; they release chemotactic factors that recruit more neutrophils. These cells release oxygen free radicals and proteolytic enzymes. Disruption of the interstitial matrix results in fluids and protein loss into the interstitial space.

TREATMENT

Treatment is designed to minimize the sequelae of pulmonary injury. Free radical scavengers should be considered, as well as the following.

Pulmonary Toilet

Chest physical therapy and postural drainage with frequent suctioning are required. Bronchoscopy is used to remove casts and debris, and brushings for culture are useful.[18]

Antibiotics

Prophylactic antibiotics do not prevent bacterial pneumonia. They can select out resistant organisms, which may predispose patients to worse pneumonia processes that are harder to eradicate. Appropriate antibiotics should be given for documented infections.

Steroids

Steroid medications reduce mucosal edema, blunt the changes in capillary permeability, and stabilize cellular membranes and lysosomes.

They may also inhibit the chemotactic action of the complement system. However, in burn patients, the side effects of these drugs outweigh the theoretical benefits. Animal models have demonstrated increased mortality in steroid-treated groups, and an increased incidence of infection. These types of complications have also been documented in adult burn patients.[19] In our unit and other units' experience, steroids are not warranted in the treatment of burn patients.

Ventilation/Oxygenation

Inverse-rate ventilation theoretically increases functional residual capacity. Mean pressures are increased without elevation of peak pressures. Pressure-control ventilation (PCV) delivers gas flow at a constant pressure. Tidal volume (VT) is determined by pressure. PCV lowers peak airway pressures and maintains minute ventilation. The pressure setting is obtained by dividing the VT by the patient's compliance.

High-frequency ventilation (HFV) has proved effective in several clinical trials in patients with isolated pulmonary injury. HFV is characterized by a ventilatory cycle of more than 60 breaths/min, lower peak airway pressures, minimal functional residual capacity (FRC), and improved clearance of bronchial secretions.[20]

Positive end-expiratory pressure (PEEP) improves oxygen saturation and reduces intrapulmonary shunting by recruiting alveoli. Providing "physiologic levels" (i.e., 5 cm H_2O) of PEEP to patients receiving ventilatory therapy is controversial. PEEP has not been shown to improve overall outcomes and has the potential to decrease cardiac output (CO) and cause barotrauma. However, oxygenation can be increased without increasing the FIO_2 to toxic levels. A "best PEEP" study can be done using the mixed venous oxygen saturation (SVO_2). The PEEP is dialed in, using this number to titrate the amount. The correct number is determined 20 minutes after each change. PEEP is also beneficial in patients who have acute respiratory distress syndrome (ARDS) and postoperative atelectasis. The beneficial effects are usually diminished with a PEEP level higher than 15 cm H$_2$O.

Other ventilatory modes include low tidal volume ventilation to decrease inspiratory pressures and further damage to the alveoli. PCV is useful when pressure and oxygenation requirements are high. Airway pressure release ventilation (APRV) applies continuous positive airway pressure (CPAP) for a prolonged time to maintain adequate lung volume and alveolar recruitment, with a time-cycled release phase to a lower set of pressure for a short period of time, where most ventilation and CO$_2$ removal occurs.[21,22] Extracorporeal membrane oxygenation (ECMO) has been used with poor results in our unit.

Ventilator Management

An understanding of the results of arterial blood gas (ABG) measurements is essential, along with the appropriate responses in the acute, posttraumatic (burn), and/or postsurgical setting.[20,23]

ABG readings typically look like this: 7.40/40/90 (pH, PCO$_2$, and PO$_2$, respectively). This is all the information needed from the ABG slip to evaluate acute respiratory processes. The information received on the ABG reading can be categorized as *oxygenation* or *ventilation*.

Oxygenation is seen in the ABG readings as the PO$_2$. There is a relationship between the PO$_2$ and the oxygen saturation (Table 7-2).

Table 7-2 The Relationship Between PO$_2$ and Oxygen Saturation

PO$_2$ (mm Hg)	O$_2$ Saturation (%)
60	90
47	75
27	50

This is expressed as the oxygen-hemoglobin dissociation curve (Fig. 7-1). Entities that move the curve to the right (offload oxygen into the bloodstream) include decreased pH, increased CO_2, increased temperature, and increased 2,3-diphosphoglycerate (2,3-DPG).

The normal relationship is reflected by these major points. Even at a PO_2 of 60 mm Hg, the saturation is still acceptable at 90%. Below this level, a steep drop-off occurs. The ABG is not needed to determine the saturation—it is already known from the PO_2. To emphasize: Only three numbers are needed from the ABG—pH, PCO_2, and PO_2.

Fig. 7-1 Oxygen-hemoglobin dissociation curve. (From Murray JF. The Normal Lung, ed 2. Philadephia: WB Saunders, 1986.)

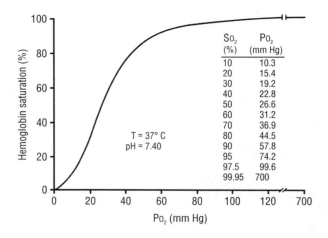

Oxygenation is managed with the ventilator, using FIO_2 and PEEP. Decreasing the FIO_2 to less than 60% is usually desirable, because higher oxygen levels are associated with toxicity to the lung tissues. There are exceptions, discussed earlier, in burn patients (e.g., carbon monoxide exposure). (See the previous discussion on PEEP.) Ventilation is managed using the minute ventilation:

Minute ventilation = Respiratory rate (RR) × Tidal volume (VT)

The clinician needs to determine whether an abnormality exists, diagnose the cause, and treat the problem. It is necessary to compute the base deficit or excess on each ABG. This is done the same way each time. In this manner, it becomes a habit, and the practitioner is less likely to "miss" abnormalities. A base deficit is also known as a *negative base excess.* The clinician should calculate the base deficit; this is more accurate than the calculation on the ABG slip. Again, only three numbers are needed on the ABG.

Determination of Base Deficit From an Arterial Blood Gas

1. A change in PCO_2 of 10 mm Hg leads to a change in the pH (in the opposite direction).

    EXAMPLE:

    a. If PCO_2 = 50 mm Hg, a decrease in the pH of 0.08 is expected. For simplicity, the PCO_2 is "up" 10 mm Hg, and the pH is "down" 8.

    b. The pH decimals are discarded, because they can be confusing.

2. Base deficit = ⅔ of the difference between predicted pH (by PCO_2 alone) and the actual pH.

    EXAMPLE: pH 7.40, PCO_2 30 mm Hg

    a. Based on the PCO_2 alone, the pH should be 7.48. The patient is "down" 10 mm Hg. Therefore the patient's pH should be "up" 8 (7.40 + 0.08 = 7.48). But he is not.

b. The measured pH from the ABG is 7.40. There is a difference between the measured and the predicted pH (7.40 and 7.48, respectively). This difference is 8 (disregarding the decimals).

c. This number (8) is multiplied by ⅔ to calculate the base deficit or excess.

$$8 \times \frac{2}{3} = 16/3, \text{ or approximately } 5$$

d. Now the pH is lower (more acidic) than expected, so there is a base deficit of 5 (or base excess of -5).

e. The threshold for a diagnosis of metabolic acidosis is usually a base deficit of 5. Acute metabolic acidosis is usually treated, with HCO_3.

Bicarbonate Replacement

1. The bicarbonate space (in liters) = $0.4 \times$ Body weight in kg $\times$ Base deficit.

   EXAMPLE: $0.4 \times 70 \text{ kg} \times 5 = 140 \text{ mEq } HCO_3$

   a. Replace HCO_3 by giving only half this amount (e.g., 70 mEq HCO_3).

   b. One ampule of HCO_3 contains 50 mEq, so the dose is 1.5 ampules.

   c. Whenever a ventilator setting is changed, HCO_3 is given, or any treatment that may affect the ventilation or acid/base status of a patient, and ABG is checked 20 minutes after the intervention. Changes in oxygenation can be assessed with the pulse oximeter, although an occasional ABG measurement may be helpful.

   d. The physician should not hesitate to increase minute ventilation to compensate for metabolic acidosis by generating a respiratory alkalosis.

  e. Generally, base deficits of greater than 5 are treated with HCO_3 replacement.

  f. Metabolic acidosis should be considered abnormal. The reason the patient is "making acid" needs to be determined and the problem treated.

2. Respiratory acidosis or alkalosis can be managed by changing the ventilator settings. As described previously, a patient with metabolic acidosis can be treated by creating a small respiratory alkalosis (on purpose).

Changing the Ventilator Setting to Change the Carbon Dioxide Level

1. PCO_2 is adjusted based on the following equation:

$$\text{Minute ventilation } (VT \times RR) = \text{Alveolar ventilation}$$

2. PCO_2 is inversely proportional to the minute ventilation (e.g., a larger minute volume will "blow off" PCO_2).

$$VT \times \text{Rate} \times CO_2 = VT \times \text{Rate} \times CO_2$$
$$\textit{Current} \qquad\qquad \textit{Desired}$$

EXAMPLE: A patient has a tidal volume of 1000 cc, a rate of 10 breaths/min, and a PCO_2 of 60 mm Hg. The goal PCO_2 is 40 mm Hg.

  a. The current numbers are placed in the following equation:

$$1000 \text{ cc } VT \times \text{Rate } 10 \text{ breaths/min} \times 60 \text{ mm Hg } CO_2$$

  b. The desired CO_2 is equal to what the clinician wants it to be: Desired CO_2 of 40

  c. The value to be changed is set equal to x (Rate $= x$ or $VT = x$). It is easier to change the rate.

$$1000 \text{ cc } VT \times \text{Rate } 10 \text{ breaths/min} \times 60 \text{ mm Hg } CO_2 =$$
$$1000 \text{ } VT \times \text{Rate } x \times 40 \text{ mm Hg } CO_2$$

d. Solve by algebra for x. This gives an estimate of the amount of change.

$$600 = 40x$$
$$15 = x$$

The rate is changed to 15 breaths/min.
  e. An ABG is obtained 20 minutes after the change to evaluate the difference.
3. The tidal volume can be changed instead of the rate if desired by solving for the tidal volume of the desired change.
4. The clinician should not "shoot from the hip" when giving HCO_3 or making ventilator changes. These tools allow accurate diagnosis and treatment. ABG is checked 20 minutes after every intervention.

EXAMPLE: A classic ABG is 7.30/35/65.

  a. The patient is "down" 5, and so should be "up" 0.04 (or rather 4). The predicted pH is 7.44. But it is not. There is a difference in the predicted and the measured pH.
  b. (7.44 predicted – 7.30 measured) = 0.14 (i.e., 14).
  c. $14 + 2/3 = 9.3$. The measured pH is more acidic than predicted. The patient has a base deficit of 9.

This patient is in *BIG TROUBLE*. He is "making" a lot of acid. The values are within the "normal" range and would not even "light up" on most ABG panels. This is the reason the base deficit needs to be computed each time ABG results are received.

The patient has metabolic acidosis. The needed amount of HCO_3 is calculated (the patient weighs 70 kg):

0.4 Bicarbonate space $\times$ 70 kg $\times$ 9 Base deficit = 252 mEq HCO_3
needed in the patient's bicarbonate space

Remember: Only half that value is given now, 126 mEq, or 2.5 ampules of HCO_3. Another ABG is checked in 20 minutes. Search for a cause.

Evaluation of Oxygenation

The patient has a PO_2 of 65 mm Hg. This should reflect a saturation of 94%. This is not a problem at this time. The PO_2 may look "low"; however, the hemoglobin-oxygen dissociation curve should be considered.

Preparing to Extubate

Patients should be able to tolerate 30 minutes of CPAP. To confirm edema is not present, the balloon on the endotracheal tube can be deflated and evaluated for an air leak. The rapid shallow breathing index is the respiratory rate divided by the tidal volume in liters. A quotient of less than 100 usually indicates the patient is ready for extubation.

USEFUL VENTILATORY EQUATIONS
A-a Gradient Equation

1. The alveolar-arterial gradient (A-a gradient) or $A-aO_2$ difference $(DA-aO_2)$ is the difference between the partial pressure of oxygen in alveoli (A) and that in arterial blood (a):

$$DA-aO_2 = PAO_2 - PaO_2$$

   a. $DA-aO_2$ is 5 to 15 mm Hg in healthy, young patients.
   b. $DA-aO_2$ is increased in all causes of hypoxemia except hypoventilation and high altitude. It increases with age and in patients with lung diseases that cause a V/Q mismatch (i.e., shunt or diffusion abnormality). A patient with a pulmonary embolus has an increased $DA-aO_2$, but if the patient is hyperventilating (as is often the case), the ABG may show a normal PaO_2.
   c. PAO_2 = Alveolar air pressure of O_2. PaO_2 = arterial air pressure of O_2. PCO_2 = Arterial air pressure of CO_2. FIO_2 = Fractional inspired oxygen.

d. To determine the $DA\text{-}aO_2$, the PaO_2 in the alveoli (PAO_2) is calculated first. This is the partial pressure of inspired O_2 minus the partial pressure of alveolar CO_2 ($PACO_2$). The $PACO_2 = PaCO_2/0.8$. The 0.8 used in this short formula represents the respiratory quotient (CO_2 produced per minute or O_2 consumed per minute). The partial pressure of CO_2 in the alveoli is slightly lower than in the arterial blood.

$$PAO_2 = \text{Inspired } PaO_2 - (PaCO_2 \div 0.8)$$

e. The inspired PaO_2 is determined by multiplying the $\%O_2$ (same as the FIO_2) (Barometric pressure $-$ Water vapor). At standard conditions, barometric pressure $= 760$ mm Hg and water vapor $= 47$ mm Hg. Plugging this back into the original formula gives:

$$DA\text{-}aO_2 = PAO_2 - PaO_2$$
$$DA\text{-}aO_2 = [FIO_2 \times (\text{Barometric pressure} - \text{Water vapor pressure}) - (PaCO_2 \div 0.8)] - PaO_2$$

Assuming standard conditions (often unlikely), the equation would be:

$$DA\text{-}aO_2 = [0.21 \times (760 - 47) - (PaCO_2 \div 0.8)] - PaO_2$$
$$DA\text{-}aO_2 = [150 - (PaCO \div 0.8)] - PaO_2$$

f. This calculation is most accurate at an FIO_2 of 0.21.
   At an FIO_2 of 0.21, normal is 10-20 mm Hg; >25 mm Hg is abnormal.
   At an FIO_2 of 1.00, >350 mm Hg is abnormal.

2. Another method to calculate this mentally at the bedside is as follows:

   a. The A-a gradient is the following:

$$DA\text{-}aO_2 = 150 - (PaO_2 + 1.25\, PaO_2)$$

    b. DA-aO$_2$ increases with age. Two rules of thumb for determining normal DA-aO$_2$ are the following:

      – Normal DA-aO$_2$ is less than or equal to $0.29 \times$ age.

      or

      – Normal DA-aO$_2$ is less than or equal to (age $\div$ 4) + 2.5.

3. Another bedside calculation is the following:

    a. The A-a gradient is: $700 \times FIO_2 - PCO_2$

    b. Abnormal is >300. *(Consider intubation.)*

4. Respiratory causes of an increased A-a gradient include diffusion barrier, right-to-left intrapulmonary shunt, and V/Q mismatch. Nonrespiratory causes include right-to-left intracardiac shunts and hyperthermia. A decreased PaO$_2$ with a normal A-a gradient is seen at high altitude, with a decreased respiratory quotient, and in central hypoventilation.

Compliance Equation

1. $C = \Delta V/\Delta P$.

2. C_{dyn} = VT/Peak transpulmonary pressure. This measures the compliance during movement of air. Desired is <0.3 cm H$_2$O/sec.

3. C_{stat} = VT/Plateau pressure = 1/Elastic recoil. This measures the compliance at end expiration, when there is no air flow. Included is the compliance of the chest wall. Normal = 0.05-0.07 L/cm H$_2$O.

REFERENCES

1. Smith DL, Cairns BA, Ramadan F, et al. Effect of inhalation injury, burn size, and age on mortality: a study of 1447 consecutive burn patients. J Trauma 37:655-659, 1994.

2. El-Helbawy RH, Ghareeb FM. Inhalation injury as a prognostic factor for mortality in burn patients. Ann Burns Fire Disasters 24:82-88, 2011.

3. Santaniello JM, Luchette FA, Esposito TJ, et al. Ten year experience of burn, trauma, and combined burn/trauma injuries comparing outcomes. J Trauma 57:696-700; discussion 700-701, 2004.

4. Rue LW III, Cioffi WG, Mason AD, et al. Improved survival of burned patients with inhalation injury. Arch Surg 128:772-778, 1993.
5. Demling R, Picard L, Campbell C, et al. Relationship of burn induced lung lipid peroxidation of the degree of injury after smoke inhalation and a body burn. Crit Care Med 21:1935-1943, 1993.
6. Chen MC, Chen MH, Wen BS, et al. The impact of inhalation injury in patients with small and moderate burns. Burns 40:1481-1486, 2014.
7. Mlcak RP, Suman OE, Herndon DN. Respiratory management of inhalation injury. Burns 33:2-13, 2007.
8. Shirani KZ, Pruitt BA Jr, Mason AD Jr. The influence of inhalation injury and pneumonia on burn mortality. Ann Surg 205:82-87, 1987.
9. Valova M, Konigova R, Broz L, et al. Early and late fatal complications of inhalation injury. Acta Chir Plast 44:51-54, 2002.
10. Einhorn IN. Physiological and toxicological aspects of smoke produced during the combustion of polymeric materials. Environ Health Perspect 11:163-189, 1975.
11. Schulte JH. Effects of mild carbon monoxide intoxication. Arch Environ Health 7:524-530, 1963.
12. Miller AC, Rivero A, Ziad S, et al. Influence of nebulized unfractionated heparin and N-acetylcysteine in acute lung injury after smoke inhalation injury. J Burn Care Res 30:249-256, 2009.
13. Miller AC, Elamin EM, Suffredini AF. Inhaled anticoagulation regimens for the treatment of smoke inhalation-associated acute lung injury: a systematic review. Crit Care Med 42:413-419, 2014.
14. Holm C, Tegeler J, Mayr M, et al. Effect of crystalloid resuscitation and inhalation injury on extravascular lung water: clinical implications. Chest 121:1956-1962, 2002.
15. American Burn Association. Pulmonary physiology and disease in the burn patient [postgraduate course]. Chicago: American Burn Association, 1996.
16. Saab M, Majid I. Acute pulmonary oedema following smoke inhalation. Int J Clin Pract 54:115-116, 2000.
17. Barillo DJ, Goode R, Esch V. Cyanide poisoning in victims of fire: analysis of 364 cases and review of the literature. J Burn Care Rehabil 15:46-51, 1994.
18. Nakae H, Tanaka H, Inaba H. Failure to clear casts and secretions following inhalation injury can be dangerous: report of a case. Burns 27:189-191, 2001.
19. Heimbach DM, Waeckerle JF. Inhalation injuries. Ann Emerg Med 17:1316-1323, 1988.
20. Derdak S. High-frequency oscillatory ventilation for accurate respiratory distress syndrome in adult patients. Crit Care Med 31(4 Suppl):S317-S323, 2003.

21. Daoud EG. Airway pressure release ventilation. Ann Thorac Med 2:176-179, 2007.
22. Downs JB, Stock MC. Airway pressure release ventilation: a new concept in ventilatory support. Crit Care Med 15:459-461, 1987.
23. Whitman GJ. Resident's Manual Cardic Surgery Service. Philadelphia: Medical College of Pennsylvania, 1994.

8 General (Nonburn) Inpatient Wound Care

KEY POINTS

- The phases of general (nonburn) inpatient wound healing are inflammatory, fibroblastic, and maturation.

- Wounds should be decontaminated to support healing, promote cleansing, decrease the bacterial count, and support epithelialization.

- Pressure sores are classified as stage I (redness), II (partial-thickness loss of skin), III (full-thickness loss of skin, exposing subcutaneous fat), and IV (full-thickness tissue loss, exposing bone, tendon, or muscle).

- A team approach is often beneficial to pressure sore prevention and treatment.

- Many factors influence wound healing, including nutrition, vascular supply, pressure, positioning, radiation, and chemotherapy.

- Venous ulcers require meticulous care.

- Diabetic foot wounds may require revascularization.

THE BASICS

Practitioners who treat patients with wounds should know the general principles of care, including the phases of wound healing, the entities that must be present, and the entities that can hamper wound healing. In this chapter we will discuss care of common and more complex wounds.

STAGES OF WOUND HEALING

The process of wound healing is categorized into various phases, which are influenced by the dominant cell type in the wound site. The phases and cell types may overlap. After the integrity of the skin is disrupted, vasoconstriction occurs and a platelet plug is formed. Platelets are essential for hemostasis; they also activate other cells and start the inflammatory cascade.

The first phase of healing is called the *lag, substrate,* or *inflammatory phase.* The wound site swells and vasodilation occurs. The reaction is mediated by multiple cytokines, growth factors, and local proteins. Some of these molecules (called *chemoattractants*) attract other cells to the wound. Leukocytes appear quickly in the wound and mediate bacterial phagocytosis and lysis. They predominate from the time of wounding until about day 3. The monocyte is the next cell type to appear; it is the key mediator of the cellular response within the wound and the predominant cell from days 3 to 7. Fibrinogen aids in adherence of the wound edges. Histamine, prostaglandins, and vasoactive substances mediate hemostasis. This phase is essential to prepare the wound for the subsequent phases of healing.

The second phase of wound healing is the *fibroblastic* or *collagen phase.* Fibroblasts begin to proliferate and prepare for their important role of collagen synthesis. They are the predominant cells in the wound. As the collagen content increases, the wound strengthens. The wound's tensile strength and collagen content increase over the next few weeks. The wound contains its maximum collagen content 6 weeks after the injury. Most remodeling is completed by 1 year after the injury; collagen turnover within the wound will continue indefinitely. The maximum bursting strength of the wound will never reach that of undamaged skin but will usually achieve 80%. This occurs by approximately 6 months after the injury.

Cofactors are important in proper collagen formation and wound healing. Ascorbic acid (vitamin C) is essential for collagen formation. Without vitamin C, proline cannot be hydroxylated to hydroxyproline, and collagen synthesis stops. Collagen resorption will continue at a normal pace, leading to scurvy. In 1747 Dr. James Lind, a surgeon in the British navy, discovered that by giving sailors limes and other citrus fruits to eat, they did not develop scurvy, thus helping to make sailors on long voyages fit for duty and earning them the nickname "limeys."

The third and final phase of wound healing lasts the longest. This is the *maturation* or *remodeling phase*. This phase may continue for several years. Progressive collagen replacement allows scars to flatten and pale with time. Most surgeons will not revise a scar until at least 9 months to 1 year after the initial injury; by this time the collagen content and remodeling usually have stabilized.[1,2]

WOUNDS WITH LOSS OF SKIN

Acute, traumatic injuries (full-thickness burn, deep abrasion, and avulsion injury) will pass through the same phases of wound healing. In such an injury, the closure and healing are more complex, requiring additional mechanisms.

Epithelial proliferation and migration are required for healing of the wound. This process starts after the biochemical and cellular milieu is ready and bacterial contamination of the wound is below 10^5 organisms per cubic centimeter of tissue. If the wound is superficial, the epithelium can spread from the sweat glands, hair follicles, and wound edges to cover the wound. Depending on its size, the wound may be covered in this fashion in 10 to 14 days. In full-thickness wounds, epithelium migrates from the wound margins.

Epithelialization is a slow process, with migration of approximately 1 mm per day. Epithelium is more susceptible to injury than the original tissue, because it migrates without an accompanying dermal layer. Histologically, migratory epithelium often appears neoplastic. A chronic wound not closed for many years may become a malignant ulcer, or *Marjolin's ulcer* (named for the French surgeon Jean-Nicolas Marjolin, who first described this entity). Therefore physicians should not wait for the wound to heal by epithelialization alone, except in very small or superficial injuries. In these cases, the wounds are covered with grafts and flaps.

Wound contraction can occur in the closure of these types of wounds. The surface fills with granulation tissue, consisting of capillary and fibroblast proliferation. After granulation occurs, myofibroblasts, behaving like smooth muscle cells, mediate the contraction of the wound. This process may lead to contractures. Contraction may be slowed by the application of split-thickness skin grafts and may be almost stopped with placement of a full-thickness skin graft.

WOUND CONTAMINATION

Contamination of the wound will stop epithelialization and contraction of the wound.[1,2] Compared with intact skin, a wound is much more susceptible to infection and breakdown. The objective in the decontamination of wounds is to reduce the bacterial count to less than 10^5 organisms per cubic centimeter of tissue. This can be accomplished with debridement of necrotic or infected tissue and irrigation. Normal saline solution is the irrigant of choice. We highly recommend that patients be given a sedative, analgesic, and a local anesthetic. Some patients require general analgesic for adequate debridement and irrigation (e.g., those with road rash after a motorcycle motor vehicle accident). Caregivers should ask patients about drug reactions and allergies and thoroughly explain the procedure.[3]

DECUBITUS ULCERS, PRESSURE SORES, AND BEDSORES

These terms describe the same entity. The word *decubitus* is from the Latin *decumbere*, meaning to lie down. The most contemporary—and accurate—term is *pressure sore*. Pressure sores are usually caused by pressure being exerted on an area of tissue, preventing adequate perfusion. These wounds can occur rapidly (in just 2 hours). Multiple factors—such as friction, sheering force, and moisture—can contribute to the development of pressure sores.

Interest has increased in the prevention, evaluation, and treatment of these wounds. They have been recognized as a significant source of morbidity and are expensive to treat. With an estimated 2.5 million pressure sores treated annually in the United States at a cost of $11 billion, pressure sores represent a costly and labor-intensive challenge to the health care system.[4,5]

Risk Factors

- *Pressure:* Causes ischemia. Muscles are more susceptible to damage (tip-of-the-iceberg effect).
- *Sheer force:* Blood vessels stretch and tear and blood flow is reduced, causing stasis and ischemic tissue necrosis.
- *Friction:* The stratum corneum (a barrier against infection) is breached.
- *Moisture:* Sweat or incontinence can break down skin.
- *Patient positioning:* Changes in body posture can generate pressure at different points in the body, making them more susceptible to pressure ulceration.
- *Immobility:* Prolonged hospital stay, bed rest, or spinal cord injury.
- *Neurologic factors:* These include sedation, weakness that decreases spontaneous movement, decreased sensation, or cognitive impairment.
- *Nutritional and metabolic factors:* These include undernutrition, with lack of calories, protein, vitamins, and trace elements.

- *Diabetes:* This can lead to anemia, peripheral arterial disease, and venous insufficiency.
- *Edema:* This decreases blood flow and oxygenation.
- *65 years of age or older:* Reduced subcutaneous fat and capillary blood flow are postulated reasons in these patients.[6,7]

Several scales have been developed to aid in the evaluation of the wound and to predict the risk for pressure sores. They include the Norton scale (Table 8-1) and the Braden scale. Both scales have been modified from the original. Some etiologic factors may not be represented in a particular scale. The use of a risk assessment scale along with skilled clinical assessment is recommended.

Assessment Using the Norton Scale

With the Norton scale, the patient is evaluated and scored in five categories: physical condition, mental condition, activity, mobility, and incontinence. The scores are totaled. Pressure sore risk increases as the score decreases. A score of less than 10 indicates a very high risk of pressure sore development. The Norton scale does not consider nutritional factors or shearing forces and does not have a functional definition of the applied parameters.

The Norton Plus scale is a modified scale in which the presence of the following are noted:

- Diabetes
- Hypertension
- Hematocrit in males $<41\%$, in females $<36\%$
- Hemoglobin in males <14 g/dl, in females <12 g/dl
- Serum albumin level <3.3 g/dl
- Fever $>37.6°$ C (99.6° F)
- Prescription medications—five or more
- Changes in mental state to confused, lethargic within 24 hours[8,9]

Once a patient is identified as being at risk, efforts must be made to treat the current issues and prevent further morbidity.

Table 8-1   The Norton Scale for Predicting Pressure Sore Risk

Criterion	Score
Physical condition	4 = Good
	3 = Fair
	2 = Poor
	1 = Very bad
Mental condition	4 = Alert
	3 = Apathetic
	2 = Confused
	1 = Stupor
Activity	4 = Ambulant
	3 = Walk with help
	2 = Chair bound
	1 = Bed bound
Mobility	4 = Full
	3 = Slightly impaired
	2 = Very limited
	1 = Immobile
Incontinent	4 = Not
	3 = Occasionally
	2 = Usually/Urine
	1 = Doubly
TOTAL	Calculated as the total of the scores in all criteria:
	Greater than 18 = Low risk
	Between 18 and 14 = Medium risk
	Between 14 and 10 = High risk
	Less than 10 = Very high risk

From Norton D, McLaren R, Exton-Smith AN. An investigation of geriatric nursing problems in hospital. London: The National Corporation for the Care of Old People, 1962.

Assessment Using the Braden Scale

The modified Braden scale is rated in several scientific journals as having the best sensitivity and specificity. This scoring system can be technically demanding, and requires some training to use it properly.

The Braden scale assesses a patient's risk of developing a pressure ulcer by examining the following six criteria[10-13]:

- *Sensory perception:* Ability to detect and respond to discomfort or pain that is related to pressure on parts of one's body.
- *Moisture:* Degree of moisture to which the skin is exposed.
- *Activity:* Level of physical activity.
- *Mobility:* Capability to adjust one's body position independently.
- *Nutrition:* Normal patterns of daily nutrition.
- *Friction and shear:* Amount of assistance one needs to move, and the degree of sliding on beds or chairs.

Scoring With the Braden Scale

Each category is rated on a scale of 1 to 4, with the exception of the 'friction and shear' category, which is rated on a scale of 1 to 3. This combines for a possible total of 23 points, with a higher score meaning a lower risk of developing a pressure sore. A score of 23 means that there is no risk for developing a pressure sore, and the lowest possible score of 6 points represents the most severe risk for developing a pressure sore.[10-13]

The Braden Scale assessment score scale is presented below[10-13]:

- Very High Risk: Total Score less than 9
- High Risk: Total Score 10-12
- Moderate Risk: Total Score 13-14
- Mild Risk: Total Score 15-18
- No Risk: Total Score 19-23

Classification of Pressure Sores

The most commonly used classification system was developed by the United States–National Pressure Ulcer Advisory Panel (US-NPUAP)[14]:

- Category/stage:
  I Redness
  II Partial-thickness loss of skin
  III Full-thickness loss of skin, exposing subcutaneous fat
  IV Full-thickness tissue loss, exposing bone, tendon, or muscle

- Additional categories/stages for the United States:
  - Suspected deep tissue injury with discolored intact skin
  - Unstageable: full-thickness tissue loss with the base covered with slough/eschar

TREATMENT
Wound Care Team

Often, practitioners who care for these wounds need to interact with other services in the hospital (e.g., plastic surgery, general surgery, nursing, physical medicine and rehabilitation, and nutrition). Organizing and working with a multidisciplinary wound care team can be a very efficient means of treatment. A team can be instrumental in decreasing the incidence and length of healing time of inpatient pressure sores, as reported in several series.[15] Wound care teams often set protocols for the proper use of appropriate beds, monitor nutritional status, and oversee other aspects of care that affect the incidence and prevalence of wounds. Their recommendations and protocols may be modified to adapt to a particular institution's needs.[16]

Unit teams can use the pathway presented in Fig. 8-1 to design a new system, as a training tool for frontline staff, and as an ongoing clinical reference tool on the units.[17] This tool can be modified or a new one created to meet the needs of a particular setting. Physicians who have prepared a process map describing their current practices can compare it with desired practices on the clinical pathway.

The principles of treatment correspond to those mentioned previously. They include good nutrition, adequate blood flow, relief from continuous pressure, relief from sheer forces, management of pain, decontamination and/or debridement of the wound, and possibly surgical coverage. Patients who are not able to move themselves should be turned every few hours and their skin inspected for signs of early breakdown.[18]

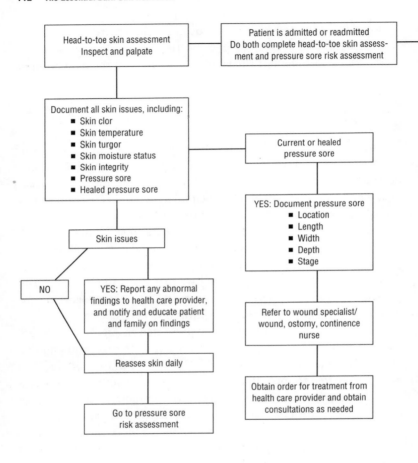

Fig. 8-1   The pathway for use by unit teams to design a new system as a training tool for frontline staff and as an ongoing clinical reference tool on the units.

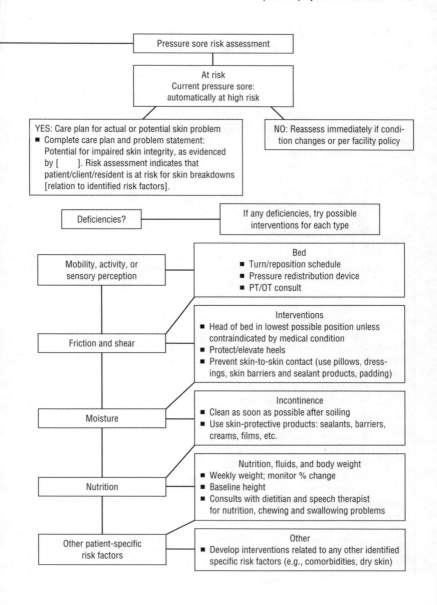

In an effort to relieve the area from continuous pressure and sheer forces, special mattresses have been devised. Criteria for their use are listed in Box 8-1.

Box 8-1
Criteria for Selection of Pressure Reduction/Relief Devices

I. Continuous airflow: Wound care committee approval required; high-risk patients with no skin breakdown

II. Low air loss: wound care committee approval required
    A. General health: Critical; major surgery with chronic/serious health problems; major/multiple injuries. Rehabilitative phase; patients whose respiratory status requires high head elevation
    B. Mental status: Comatose; minimal/no verbal response; minimal/no motor response to painful stimuli
    C. Activity: Patients requiring transfer; completely bedridden
    D. Mobility: Very limited or immobile; minimal voluntary movement/positioning
    E. Elimination: Frequent/complete loss of bowel and bladder control; signs of maceration from exposure to urine/feces
    F. Nutrition: Consumes 50% of recommended diet; orally or intravenously only; albumin 2.5 g/dl.
    G. Skin integrity: Stage II; noninfected stages III and IV

III. Air fluidized: Wound care committee approval required
    A. General health: Critical; major surgery with chronic/serious health problems; major/multiple injuries. Burn patients; patients with skin grafts, flaps, donor sites; multiple trauma in acute phase
    B. Mental status: Comatose; minimal/no verbal response; minimal/no motor response to painful stimuli
    C. Activity: Completely bedridden
    D. Mobility: Immobile; minimal to no voluntary movement/positioning
    E. Elimination: Frequent/complete loss of bowel and bladder control; signs of maceration from exposure to urine/feces
    F. Nutrition: Consumes 50% of recommended diet; orally or intravenously only; albumin 2.5 g/dl
    G. Skin integrity: Complicated stage II; stages III and IV and multiple pressure sores

From Granick MS, Solomon MP, Wind S, et al. Wound care and wound management. In Habal MB, Lineaweaver W, Parsons RW, et al, eds. Advances in Plastic and Reconstructive Surgery, vol 12, St Louis: Mosby–Year Book, 1996.

A modified Norton scale bed is indicated when one or more apply, when individual patient treatment objectives are considered.

Debridement

The principles of debridement of these wounds are discussed in Chapter 5. Sharp debridement of necrotic, infected, or fibrous tissue may be necessary. This usually can be performed at the patient's bedside. Debridement with the use of dressings may be appropriate in some cases to keep the wound clean. Wet-to-dry dressings with normal saline solution, changed three times per day, will debride small amounts of material. Dakin's solution, a 1:1000 mixture of povidone-iodine and saline solution, or 0.5% acetic acid in saline solution may be used if bacterial overgrowth is suspected. Wet dressings should not be applied to nonwounded skin.[19-22]

Granulation tissue, normally a welcome entity in wound healing, may occasionally be too productive and hamper the epithelialization process. The use of silver nitrate sticks can decrease the amount of granulation tissue to allow epithelialization.

Table 8-2 is a guide to wound care objectives and the products used to achieve them.

Negative Pressure Wound Therapy

Negative pressure wound therapy (NPWT) devices have made a tremendous impact on the inpatient (and now outpatient) management of wounds. This modality is useful in many cases to help contract the wound and to keep it clean. Fewer dressing changes are involved, easing the burden on the nursing staff and the patient. Fewer hands treating the wound has been postulated to decrease the risk of contamination. With NPWT, wounds can be treated while patients are given nutritional support, improving the nutritional status for wound healing. The size of the wound is often decreased, allowing a less sophisticated method of surgical coverage.[23,24] Treatment may increase

Text continued on p. 121.

Table 8-2 Wound Care Products by Objective

Wound Care Objective	Product		Function	Outcome	Cautions	Example (Manufacturer)
	Category					
Cleansing						
Skin	Liquid/foam skin		Emulsifies waste materials, neutralizes drainage and odors	Facilitates the removal of surface debris	Use *around* wounds, not for use *in* wounds	CarraFoam (Carrington) Bedside-Care Perineal Wash (Coloplast) Triple Care (Smith & Nephew)
Wound	Absorbent foam					
	Hydrophilic-hydrophobic		Absorption of minimal to heavy exudate, nonadherent	Nonadherent, decreased tissue trauma on removal	Affixed by external dressing, do not allow to dry out	Allevyn (Smith & Nephew) Epi-Lock (Calgon Vestal) Lyofoam (Mölnlycke Health Care)
	Gels		Absorb minimal to heavy exudate, soften necrotic tissue, nonadherent	Conforms to wound surface, eliminates dead space, moist environment	Requires cover dressing, replace as needed to keep wound base moist	Absorption Dressing (Bard) Intrasite (Smith & Nephew) Hypergel (Mölnlycke Health Care)
	Hydrogels		Absorb minimal exudate, nonadherent, may soften necrosis	Creates moist environment, soothes and protects	Do not allow to dry out, may require cover dressing to hold in place	Aquasorb (DeRoyal) Nu-Gel (Johnson & Johnson) Vigilon (Bard)

	Normal saline solution, sprays	Mechanical cleansing action—sometimes used to "wet" dressings	Removes surface debris without wound irritation	Do not apply with excessive force	Dermal Wound Cleansers (Smith & Nephew) Puri-Clens (Sween Inc.) Shur-Clens (ConvaTec; Bristol-Myers Squibb) Mesalt (Scott Health Care)
	Impregnated gauze Crystalline sodium chloride dressing	Osmotic action "wicks" exudate from wound and surrounding tissue	Cleanses and reduces edema, retards bacterial growth	Cover with dry dressing to absorb exudate	
Autolytic	Hydrocolloids	Occlusion traps exudate, helps white blood cells to liquefy and phagocytize necrosis	Selective (specific) debridement, some absorption of exudate	Never use on any wound suspected of being infected	Duoderm (ConvaTec; Bristol-Myers Squibb) Restore (Hollister) Replicare (Smith & Nephew) Tegasorb (3M)
	Hydrogels	Moisture helps soften eschar in dry, necrotic wounds	Softens and aids removal of eschar	Held in place by external dressing, do not allow to dry out	Aquasorb (DeRoyal Industries) Hypergel (Mölnlycke Health Care) Nu-Gel (Johnson & Johnson) SoloSite (Smith & Nephew)
	MVP films, semi-occlusive	Acts as occlusive, also allows the exchange of gases, vapors	Selective debridement	Do not use on infected wounds	Bioclusive (Johnson & Johnson) OpSite (Smith & Nephew) Tegaderm (3M)

From Granick MS, Solomon MP, Wind S, et al. Wound care and wound management. In Habal MB, Lineaweaver W, Parsons RW, et al, eds. Advances in Plastic and Reconstructive Surgery, vol 12, St Louis: Mosby–Year Book, 1996.

Continued

Table 8-2 Wound Care Products by Objective—cont'd

Wound Care Objective	Product Category	Function	Outcome	Cautions	Example (Manufacturer)
Cleansing—cont'd					
Chemical	Enzymes	Chemically digest debris and necrotic tissue	Nonselective (nonspecific) debridement	Cross hatch eschar, protect peri-wound; iodine renders some ineffective	Collagenase (Santyl; Smith & Nephew) Fibrinolysin (Elase; Pfizer) Sutilains (Travase; Flint)
Mechanical	Impregnated gauze Crystalline sodium chloride dressing	Creates hypertonic environment, "wicks" bacteria, softens necrotic tissue	Selective debridement	Cover with dry dressings to absorb exudate	Mesalt (Scott Health Care)
	Surgical	Dissection	Selective debridement	Wound increases in size	
	Wet-to-dry	Plain gauze traps wound debris	Nonselective debridement	Not for patients with bleeding problems	Nu-Brede (Johnson & Johnson)
	Whirlpool/irrigations	Mechanical removal of debris, necrosis	Nonselective debridement	Force rather than solution gives results	

Protection

Skin	Creams, lotions, ointments, sprays	Lubricates, softens, some form occlusive barrier	Rehydration and/or protection	Predominantly used on intact skin	Moisture Barrier Ointment (Carrington) Peri-care (Sween Inc.) Moisture Barrier (Coloplast) Triple Care (Smith & Nephew) Uni-salve (Smith & Nephew)
	Skin sealants	Forms layer of plastic polymer over skin	Protection from corrosive drainage and friction of tape removal	May contain varying amounts of alcohol that stings denuded skin	Allkare (ConvaTec; Bristol-Myers Squibb) Protective Barrier Film (Bard) Skin Gel (Hollister) Skin Prep (Smith & Nephew)
Wound	MVP films, semiocclusive	Forms semiocclusive seal over wound	Protection, moist wound base	*Never* use on infected wound	Bioclusive (Johnson & Johnson) OpSite (Smith & Nephew) Tegaderm (3M)
	Foam dressings, semiocclusive	Forms semiocclusive seal over wound; reportedly maintains wound temperature	Protects, provides moist wound base	Must be affixed by external dressing	Alevyn (Smith & Nephew) Epi-Lock (Calgon Vestal) Lyofoam (Mölnlycke Health Care)

Continued

Table 8-2 Wound Care Products by Objective—cont'd

Wound Care Objective	Product		Function	Outcome	Cautions	Example (Manufacturer)
	Category					
Protection— cont'd						
Wound— cont'd	Gelatin/pectin wafers (occlusive)		Forms occlusive seal, absorbs skin moisture to prevent maceration	Protection, moist wound base	*Never* use on infected wound	Premium Barrier (Hollister) Stomahesive (ConvaTec; Bristol-Myers Squibb) Sween-A-Peel (Sween Inc.)
	Hydrocolloids (occlusive)		As gelatin, forms gel over wound bed to decrease trauma of removal	Protection, moist wound base, less removal trauma	*Never* use on infected wound	DuoDerm (ConvaTec; Bristol-Myers Squibb) Replicare (Smith & Nephew) Restore (Hollister) Tegasorb (3M)
	Ointments, gels		Provides protective, moist environment	Moist wound base	Reapply often to maintain moist environment	Biolex Wound Gel (Bard) Dermal Wound Gel (Carrington) Dermagram (Derma Sciences)

vascularized granulation tissue in the wound bed, which often can improve skin graft take.[19-25] NPWT is increasingly the modality of choice. One study suggests that the material used as the dressing (reticulated open cell foam versus gauze) and the pressure used have a significant effect on cellular response.[26] More recently, the closed NPWT system has been modified to allow irrigation through the wound bed. Several studies have shown a benefit.[19,20,22,27,28] Studies continue to determine whether this is a significant advantage to wound healing and in which wounds this adaptation may be most appropriate.[29]

Surgical Coverage

Various surgical procedures can benefit patients with significant wounds. Myocutaneous flaps and skin grafts are appropriate in selected patients.[30,31] The underlying principles include coverage of vital structures, restoration of function and form, and a decreased burden of healing for large wounds. Another principle is to attempt to use the least invasive method to obtain the desired result. A caveat when discussing wound coverage is that a free tissue transfer, although more sophisticated, may be the best option in some cases.[32]

Prognosis

The prognosis for early-stage pressure sores is excellent, with timely, appropriate treatment, but healing typically requires weeks. After 6 months of treatment, more than 70% of stage II, 50% of stage III, and 30% of stage IV wounds resolve.[6] Stage III and IV lesions may take months to heal and often require surgical intervention. Pressure sores often develop in patients who cannot be medically optimized or cannot obtain reasonable care. If these issues cannot be improved, the long-term outcome is poor, even if short-term wound healing is successful.[5]

OTHER WOUND ISSUES
Infected Wounds

Infected wounds should be left open until contamination and infection are controlled and the normal wound-healing process begins. Identification and treatment of the infectious cause depends on appropriate antibiotics, irrigation, and debridement to resolve the problem. Myocutaneous flaps may be used in some cases to bring coverage and a blood supply to the debrided area.[31,33,34]

Tissue Damage From Radiotherapy

Radiotherapy can be an important adjunct in the treatment of cancer. Radiation kills tumor cells but damages normal surrounding tissues. The amount of injury depends on a cell's susceptibility to radiation, its stage in the growth cycle, and its growth rate. Radiation damage to the skin in the acute phase is secondary to an inflammatory reaction, causing the skin to be dry, erythematous, and scaly. These acute side effects usually resolve within 6 months. Chronic side effects that appear later (beyond 6 months) are atrophy, edema, hyperpigmentation or hypopigmentation, fissuring, brittleness, and telangiectasias. Delayed complications of radiotherapy include spontaneous necrosis, the inability of wounds to heal, alteration of the local blood supply, fibrosis, and secondary tumors.[35-37]

Radiotherapy is reported to have its maximal effect on wound healing when given within 2 weeks of surgery. Injury to fibroblasts and endothelial cells and decreased collagen production are thought to account for some of the mechanisms causing impaired wound healing. Fibrosis of blood vessels, leading to impaired perfusion and lower percutaneous oxygen tension within the wound tissue, has also been implicated. Some suggest that radiotherapy be withheld until 2 to 3 weeks after surgery, at which time initial wound healing may be completed.[38-41]

When a patient develops skin breakdown within a zone of irradiated tissue, a biopsy should be performed to rule out tumor recurrence or secondary tumor. Local management of the wound requires aggressive debridement of all devitalized tissue, including skeletal support when necessary. Vascularized nonirradiated tissue is often required for adequate reconstruction.[30,42]

Chemotherapy

It may be prudent to delay chemotherapy until 7 to 10 days after surgery.[43] Chemotherapeutic agents may hamper growth factors and other mechanisms engaged in healing the wound.[37] Many products of oncogenes are similar, if not identical, to growth factors. Many schemas of cancerous replication are similar to those in wound repair. The use of topical growth factors is contraindicated in most cancerous wounds.[44]

Leg Ulcerations
VENOUS STASIS

Chronic venous disease is a prominent cause of leg ulcers. Venous ulcerations can also be caused by phlebitic syndromes, chronic venous stasis, and deep venous thrombosis. Venous ulcers are typically located on the medial malleolar area and are usually superficial with a good bed of granulation tissue. The limbs are often edematous and indurated, with considerable chronic skin atrophy.

Patients with diabetes frequently develop distal neuropathies that lead to ulceration. These individuals' altered sensation can allow ulcers on the lower extremities to go unnoticed until the wounds become advanced. In addition, these wounds often become secondarily infected.

Conservative treatment of venous ulcers involves local treatment and compression therapy. Surgical treatment is based on correction of venous hypertension and treatment of incompetent superficial, deep, and perforating veins. The addition of surgical treatment (superficial and perforating vein surgery) in appropriately selected patients with venous ulceration disease can significantly increase a patient's chance of being ulcer free, compared with ambulatory compression therapy alone. This effect was shown to persist after 10 years of follow-up.[45] The number of incompetent perforating veins has a significant effect on the ulcer state and recurrence. Research into other therapeutic strategies continues.[46]

PERIPHERAL VASCULAR DISEASE

Peripheral vascular disease of the lower extremities is a known risk factor for delayed wound healing, with an increasing propensity for ulceration, infection, and gangrene. Associated risk factors include those that lead to atherosclerosis (e.g., cigarette smoking, hypertension, hyperlipidemia, and diabetes mellitus).

Less commonly, leg ulcerations are caused by other diseases, such as rheumatoid arthritis, ankylosing spondylitis, and sickle cell disease, or are the result of an underlying squamous or basal cell carcinoma.

The treatment of leg ulcers depends on an adequate blood supply. Once this is ensured by medical treatment (with appropriate medicines) and/or surgical modalities (i.e., vascular bypass) and the patient's status has been medically optimized (i.e., cardiopulmonary maximization and/or negative pressure application to the wound), reconstruction with the use of grafts or flaps can be considered if necessary.[30,38,47]

REFERENCES

1. Verheyden CN, Losee J, Miller MJ, et al, eds. Plastic and Reconstructive Surgery: Essentials for Students, ed 6. Arlington Heights, IL: Plastic Surgery Educational Foundation, 2002.
2. Simmons RL, Steed DL. Wound healing. In Simmons RL, Steed DL, Simmons J, eds. Basic Science Review for Surgeons. Philadelphia: WB Saunders, 1992.
3. Fisher JC, Achauer BM, Brody GS, et al, eds. Everyday Wounds: A Guide for the Primary Care Physician. Arlington Heights, IL: Plastic Surgery Educational Foundation, 1997.
4. Levine SM, Sinno S, Levine JP, et al. An evidence-based approach to the surgical management of pressure ulcers. Ann Plast Surg 69:482-484, 2012.

5. Cushing CA, Phillips LG. Evidence-based medicine: pressure sores. Plast Reconstr Surg 132:1720-1732, 2013.
6. The Merck Manual, Professional Edition. Whitehouse Station, NJ: Merck Sharp & Dohme Corp, 2015.
7. Agrawal K, Chauhan N. Pressure ulcers: back to the basics. Indian J Plast Surg 45:244-254, 2012.
8. Gosnell DJ. An assessment tool to identify pressure sores. Nurs Res 22:55-59, 1973.
9. Berglund B, Nordström G. The use of the Modified Norton Scale in nursing-home patients. Scand J Caring Sci 9:165-169, 1995.
10. Berman A, Snyder S, Kozier B, et al. Kozier and Erb's Fundamentals of Nursing: Concepts, Process, and Practice, ed 8. Upper Saddle River, NJ: Prentice Hall, 2008.
11. US National Library of Medicine. 2012AA Braden scale source information, 2013. Available at *http://www.nlm.nih.gov/research/umls/sourcereleasedocs/current/LNC_BRADEN/*.
12. Osuala EO. Innovation in prevention and treatment of pressure ulcer: nursing implications. Tropical Journal of Medical Research 17:61-68, 2014.
13. US Department of Health and Human Services, Panel for the Prediction and Prevention of Pressure Ulcers in Adults. Pressure ulcers in adults: prediction and prevention. Clinical Practice Guideline, No. 3, May 1992.
14. The National Pressure Ulcer Advisor Panel. NPUAP pressure ulcer stages/categories. Available at *http://www.npuap.org/resources/educational-and-clinical-resources/npuap-pressure-ulcer-stagescategories/*.
15. Granick MS, Solomon MP, Wind S, et al. Wound management and wound care. Adv Plast Reconstr Surg 12:99-121, 1996.
16. Granick MS, Long CD. Outcome assessment of an in-hospital cross-functional wound care team. Plast Reconstr Surg 113:671-672, 2004.
17. Niederhauser A, VanDeusen Lukas C, Parker V, et al. Comprehensive programs for preventing pressure ulcers: a review of the literature. Adv Skin Wound Care 25:167-188, 2012.
18. Banks MD, Graves N, Bauer JD, et al. Cost effectiveness of nutrition support in the prevention of pressure ulcer in hospitals. Eur J Clin Nutr 67:42-46, 2013.
19. Raad W, Lantis JC II, Tyrie L, et al. Vacuum-assisted closure instill as a method of sterilizing massive venous stasis wounds prior to split thickness skin graft placement. Int Wound J7:81-85, 2010.
20. Jeong HS, Lee BH, Lee HK, et al. Negative pressure wound therapy of chronically infected wounds using 1% acetic acid irrigation. Arch Plast Surg 42:59-67, 2015.
21. Kumara DU, Fernando SS, Kottahachchi J, et al. Evaluation of bactericidal effect of three antiseptics on bacteria isolated from wounds. J Wound Care 24:5-10, 2015.

22. Back DA, Scheuermann-Poley C, Willy C. Recommendations on negative pressure wound therapy with instillation and antimicrobial solutions—when, where and how to use: what does the evidence show? Int Wound J 10(Suppl 1):S32-S42, 2013.

23. Ford CN, Reinhard ER, Yeh D, et al. Interim analysis of a prospective, randomized trial of vacuum-assisted closure versus the healthpoint system in the management of pressure ulcers. Ann Plast Surg 49:55-61, 2002.

24. Niezgoda JA, Mendez-Eastman S. The effective management of pressure ulcers. Adv Skin Wound Care 19(Suppl 1):S3-S15, 2006.

25. Yang CK, Alcantara S, Goss S, et al. Cost analysis of negative-pressure wound therapy with instillation for wound bed preparation preceding split-thickness skin grafts for massive (>100 cm^2) chronic venous leg ulcers. J Vasc Surg 61:995-999, 2015.

26. McNulty AK, Schmidt M, Feeley T, et al. Effects of negative pressure wound therapy on cellular energetics in fibroblasts grown in a provisional wound (fibrin) matrix. Wound Repair Regen 17:192-199, 2009.

27. Kim PJ, Attinger CE, Steinberg JS, et al. Negative-pressure wound therapy with instillation: international consensus guidelines. Plast Reconstr Surg 132:1569-1579, 2013.

28. Gabriel A, Kahn K, Karmy-Jones R. Use of negative pressure wound therapy with automated, volumetric instillation for the treatment of extremity and trunk wounds: clinical outcomes and potential cost-effectiveness. Eplasty 14:e41, 2014.

29. Gabriel A. Integrated negative pressure wound therapy system with volumetric automated fluid instillation in wounds at risk for compromised healing. Int Wound J 9(Suppl 1):S25-S31, 2012.

30. Foster RD, Anthony JP, Mathes SJ, et al. Flap selection as a determinant of success in pressure sore coverage. Arch Surg 132:868-873, 1997.

31. Anthony JP, Huntsman WT, Mathes SJ. Changing trends in the management of pelvic pressure ulcers: a 12-year review. Decubitus 5:44-47, 50-51, 1992.

32. He J, Xu H, Wang T, et al. Treatment of complex ischial pressure sores with free partial lateral latissimus dorsi musculocutaneous flaps in paraplegic patients. J Plast Reconstr Aesthet Surg 65:634-639, 2012.

33. Hughes T, Yu JT, Wong KY, et al. "Emergency" definitive reconstruction of a necrotising fasciitis thigh debridement defect with a pedicled TRAM flap. Int J Surg Case Rep 4:453-455, 2013.

34. Shih PK, Cheng HT, Wu CI, et al. Management of infected groin wounds after vascular surgery. Surg Infect (Larchmt) 14:325-330, 2013.

35. Mendelsohn FA, Divino CM, Reis ED, et al. Wound care after radiation therapy. Adv Skin Wound Care 15:216-224, 2002.

36. Moore J, Isler M, Barry J, et al. Major wound complication risk factors following soft tissue sarcoma resection. Eur J Surg Oncol 40:1671-1676, 2014.
37. Drake DB, Oishi SN. Wound healing considerations in chemotherapy and radiation therapy. Clin Plast Surg 22:31-37, 1995.
38. McCaw DL. The effects of cancer and cancer therapies on wound healing. Semin Vet Med Surg Small Anim 4:281-286, 1989.
39. National Cancer Intelligence Network (NCIN) Data Briefing. Time from final surgery to radiotherapy for screen-detected breast cancers. NCIN, 2012.
40. Mendelsohn FA, Divino CM, Reis ED, et al. Wound care after radiation therapy. Adv Skin Wound Care 15:216-224, 2002.
41. Payne WG, Naidu DK, Wheeler CK, et al. Wound healing in patients with cancer. Eplasty 8:e9, 2008.
42. Schwartz A, Rebecca A, Smith A, et al. Risk factors for significant wound complications following wide resection of extremity soft tissue sarcomas. Clin Orthop Relat Res 471:3612-3617, 2013.
43. Falcone RE, Nappi JF. Chemotherapy and wound healing. Surg Clin North Am 64:779-794, 1984.
44. Roth JJ, Albo D, Rothman VL, et al. Thrombospondin-1 and its CSVTCG-specific receptor in wound healing and cancer. Ann Plast Surg 40:494-501, 1998.
45. van Gent W, Catarinella F, Lam Y, et al. Conservative versus surgical treatment of venous leg ulcers: 10-year follow up of a randomized, multicenter trial. Phlebology 30(1 Suppl):S35-S41, 2015.
46. Kirsner RS, Baquerizo Nole KL, Fox JD, et al. Healing refractory venous ulcers: new treatments offer hope. J Invest Dermatol 135:19-23, 2015.
47. Lau HC, Granick MS, Aisner AM, et al. Wound care in the elderly patient. Surg Clin North Am 74:441-463, 1994.

Toxic Epidermal Necrolysis Syndrome and Stevens-Johnson Syndrome

---

KEY POINTS

- Toxic epidermal necrolysis syndrome (TENS) is a severe allergic reaction that carries a high mortality rate.

- TENS patients with large wounds often benefit from care in the burn unit.

- Other disease processes must be ruled out.

- Steroids and antibiotics are stopped on admission, unless a specific infection is being treated.

- The mortality from SCORTEN is discussed with the patient and the family.

- Care is mostly supportive until the patient heals.

In 1956 Dr. Alan Lyell, a Scottish dermatologist, described what he called *toxic epidermal necrolysis syndrome* (TENS) in four patients who "looked as though they had been scalded, but there was no history of any burn."[1] Lyell described this as an "exanthematic eruption followed by generalized exfoliation" and thought that it was caused by an unidentified toxin, causing necrosis and epidermolysis. As more patients presented with this disease, it became more apparent that it was drug induced. Some still refer to the disease as *Lyell syndrome*.

Stevens-Johnson syndrome (SJS) was first described in two young boys in 1922 as an acute mucocutaneous syndrome. Clinical findings included severe purulent conjunctivitis, severe stomatitis with extensive mucosal necrosis, and purpuric nodules. Later, this disease was noted to be drug induced in most cases.

The current thinking is that TENS and SJS are on a spectrum of severe epidermolytic adverse cutaneous drug reactions. They are distinguished by the extent of skin detachment. SJS is defined as skin detachment of 10% or less, whereas TENS is defined as skin detachment of 30% or more. Patients with skin detachment between the two standards are considered to be in an overlap group.[2]

TENS and SJS should be distinguished from erythema multiforme major (EM). Studies suggest that they are distinct disorders.[3-5]

TENS/SJS is a rare, life-threatening disease usually caused by a reaction to a drug. The disease causes the epidermis to detach from the dermis. This can happen throughout the body, leaving the patient susceptible to infection and sepsis. The mortality rate is commonly stated to be 25% to 30%. Death usually results from sepsis and subsequent multiorgan system failure. TENS/SJS has an incidence of 2 in 1 million. Some disease entities make patients more susceptible (e.g., HIV patients are 1000 times more likely to acquire the disease, with an incidence of 1:1000). Other factors can include some human leukocyte antigen (HLA) types, cancer, and subsequent radiotherapy.[6]

TENS/SJS is usually a drug-induced, dose-independent reaction. Drugs are reported to cause 80% to 95% of TENS/SJS cases. The sulfonamides and phenytoin are classically recognized as the most common etiologic agents.[7] Many drugs have been associated with TENS/SJS.

Common drugs include the following:

- Allopurinol
- Antibiotics
  - Sulfonamides (sulfamethazole, sulfadiazine, and sulfapyridine)
  - Beta-lactams (cephalosporins, penicillins [notably ampicillin], and carbapenems)
- Anticonvulsants (phenobarbitol, phenytoin, carbamazepine, and valproate)
- Antimetabolites (methotrexate)
- Antiretrovirals
- Corticosteroids
- NSAIDs (notably piroxicam and meloxicam)
- Quinalones

TENS/SJS develops approximately 1 to 3 weeks after the drug is given. However, this period can be up to 8 weeks after phenytoin is given. If the patient has had a previous reaction to the drug, the period can be as short as 2 days. In addition to drugs, other factors associated with TENS/SJS include infection with *Mycoplasma pneumoniae*, dengue virus, and cytomegalovirus; contrast agents; bone marrow and organ transplants; and malignancies.

PATHOPHYSIOLOGY

The pathophysiology of TENS/SJS is poorly understood. Most think the cause is immunologic. The presentation is similar to that of a hypersensitivity reaction. It has a delayed reaction to an initial exposure, and an increasingly swift reaction with repeated exposure. It is thought to be a cytotoxic reaction aimed at destroying keratinocytes that express a foreign antigen. Keratinocytes are found in the basal layer (stratum basale) of the skin. They make up 90% of the cells of the epidermis and hold the surrounding skin cells together. It seems that CD8+ T cells become overactive by stimulation from drugs or drug metabolites. The CD8+ T cells then mediate keratinocyte cell death through release of a number of molecules, including perforin, granzyme B, and granulysin.[3] Other agents, including tumor necrosis factor–alpha (TNF-a) and Fas ligand, also appear to be involved in TENS/SJS pathogenesis. Monocellular infiltrates are often detected in the dermis. Lymphokine involvement may also mediate the epidermal injury.[8] Some patients (notably Han Chinese) have a genetic predisposition.[9]

CLINICAL PRESENTATION

The clinical presentation of TENS/SJS begins with a prodrome of fever and other symptoms that resemble an upper respiratory tract infection (i.e., fever, rhinorrhea, cough, malaise, and decreased appetite). This can continue for 1 to 3 weeks before cutaneous involvement is noted. The patient demonstrates fever and sloughing of the epidermis and mucous membranes. Then this acute cutaneous phase can last for 1 to 2 weeks. Urticarial plaques are typically present; these progress to bullae and coalesce. The fluid within them is clear, yellow, and acellular. The epidermis will slough in large sheets, denuding the dermis. A *Nikolsky sign* (in which an eraser is placed gently on the skin and twirled back and forth) is often present but can be nonspecific. If the test result is positive, a blister will form in the area, usually within minutes. An *Asboe-Hanson sign* (in which pressure placed on a bulla causes it to extend laterally) may also be present but can be nonspecific. These signs show that the top layers of the skin will slip away from the lower layers. The dislodgement of intact superficial epidermis by a shearing force indicates a plane of cleavage in the skin.[6]

One in seven patients will lose 100% of the epidermis. The scalp is the only area where this process does not seem to occur. Any other epidermal surface can be involved. Commonly, TENS/SJS patients have oral, ocular, and genital involvement. Oral involvement may include painful blisters that necessitate placement of an NGT or a G tube for enteral feedings. Ocular symptoms can include swelling, crusting, and ulcerations. Severe conjunctivitis is common. Blindness is possible.[10,11]

Less often, other mucosal surfaces such as the gastrointestinal tract (including the gallbladder and pancreas) are involved. The disease can involve the respiratory tract and the vaginal membranes.

TENS/SJS carries a high morbidity rate. This can be secondary to respiratory or renal failure, gastrointestinal bleeding, pulmonary embolism, and sepsis.[12] Mortality rates are also significant; sepsis is the most common cause of death in TENS/SJS patients. *Pseudomonas* and *Staphylococcus* are the most commonly identified organisms.

Recovery time is usually 1 to 2 weeks. TENS/SJS injury typically heals more rapidly than burned skin. The healing process will be slowed by infection, trauma, and pressure.

PROGNOSIS

The SCORe of Toxic Epidermal Necrolysis (SCORTEN) scale is a severity-of-illness scale that helps to predict a patient's mortality. It is based on seven independent risk factors:

1. Age: >40 years
2. Associated malignancy
3. Heart rate (beats/min): >120
4. Serum BUN (mg/dl): >27
5. Detached or compromised body surface: >10%
6. Serum bicarbonate (mEq/L): <20
7. Serum glucose (mg/dl): >250

The more risk factors present, the higher the SCORTEN score, and the higher the mortality rate[13] (Table 9-1).

Table 9-1   Mortality Rates and SCORTEN Score Results

Number of Risk Factors	Mortality Rate (%)
0-1	3.2
2	12.1
3	35.3
4	58.3
5 or more	>90

Data from Bastuji-Garin S, Fouchard N, Bertocchi M, et al. SCORTEN: a severity-of-illness score for toxic epidermal necrolysis. J Invest Dermatol 115:149-153, 2000.

DIFFERENTIAL DIAGNOSIS
Erythema Multiforme Major

A large prospective study recently stated that *erythema multiforme major* (EM) differs from SJS and TENS not only in severity, but also in several demographic characteristics and causes. EM occurs more often in younger males, with less fever, more frequent recurrences, and milder mucosal lesions. It does not seem to be associated with collagen vascular diseases, HIV infection, or cancer. Recent or recurrent herpes has been reported to be the principal risk factor for EM (29% and 17%, respectively) and has a role in SJS (6% and 10%, respectively), but not in TENS. Drugs have been found to be a more common cause of SJS and TENS (64% to 66%) than of EM (18%).[4,13]

Staphylococcal Scalded Skin Syndrome and Ritter Disease

Staphylococcal scalded skin syndrome (SSSS) is caused by certain *S. aureus* strains. It is toxin mediated (as opposed to TENS/SJS, which is usually drug induced). In SSSS, the serine proteases are spread by the circulation and can cause widespread epidermal damage at distant sites. The superficial epidermis becomes detached. TENS/SJS and SSSS can be differentiated by a biopsy examination. Patients with

TENS/SJS have full-thickness epidermal detachment and sloughing with full-thickness epidermal necrosis. SSSS is a disease characterized by red, blistered skin that resembles a burn or a scald. It typically affects neonates and children younger than 5 years of age, but can occur in predisposed adults. Ninety-eight percent of cases occur in children younger than 6 years of age. The incidence is estimated to be 0.09 to 0.13 cases per million people.[14,15]

TREATMENT OF TOXIC EPIDERMAL NECROLYSIS AND STEVENS-JOHNSON SYNDROME

Early identification and early cessation of the causative drug, when possible, are associated with better outcomes. Most treatment modalities involve intensive supportive care and early recognition of sequelae. Fluid and electrolyte, nutrition, and infection status require careful monitoring and appropriate, timely intervention.

The burn center is an ideal place for the treatment of TENS/SJS patients.[7,16-18] Staff members are well trained and comfortable treating patients with massive cutaneous injuries and the concomitant systemic effects. The physical plant is conducive to the specialized treatment needed and the measures to bring comfort to these patients.

On admission to the burn unit, steroidal medications are discontinued because of the increased morbidity and mortality rate associated with their use. An eosinophil count is obtained. An elevation usually shows that the previously given drug is being released from storage in the body's cells. Oral steroids are given to help regulate tapering of the steroidal agent.

Systemic antibiotics are discontinued if the patient has no signs of sepsis and no documented infection. The patient's blood, urine, and sputum cultures are sent at the time of admission and every 3 to 4 days thereafter. Indwelling catheters are removed or changed. If the patient is evolving on admission, a single dose of parental steroids may be given. The benefits are uncertain, however; some patients on steroids have continued to develop lesions. Fluid resuscitation is important. Less fluid is needed than is typical in burn resuscitation, because less edema forms in TENS/SJS patients.

The burn team should remove loose epidermis and send a biopsy sample for confirmation of the diagnosis. Porcine xenografts are used for coverage. The face is covered with bacitracin; silver nitrate is applied to areas not covered by xenografts. Silver sulfadiazine and mafenide are not used, because they have been known to cause TENS/SJS.

TENS/SJS can permanently damage vision. The ophthalmology service should be consulted early in the course of treatment for a TENS/SJS patient.[19] Antibiotic solutions are given to treat conjunctivitis. Adhesions can form on the conjunctival surfaces. These should be brushed aside with a glass rod up to four times per day to prevent immobilization. Warm compresses and rinses with saline solution may relieve discomfort. Patients can wear dark glasses to relieve photophobia.

Nutrition is important in the treatment of these patients. They have nitrogen loss and an increased metabolic rate. Usually 2500 kcal/day will provide sufficient calories; this is a starting point. The patient's nutritional status should be monitored (see Chapter 6). Enteral feeding is the preferred route for patients who can tolerate it. Procalamine can be given to augment the patient's intake through a peripheral intravenous line. If this is not sufficient, triphosphopyridine nucleotide through a central line should be considered.

Improved treatment techniques and critical care have decreased the mortality and morbidity from TENS/SJS. Prompt recognition of the disease and admission of the patient to an appropriate care center—the burn unit, with its previously mentioned attributes—have aided in the treatment of adults and children.[18,20-23]

Research continues in the pathophysiology and treatment of this disease. One promising treatment for TENS/SJS is immunoglobulin.[24-26] Cyclosporine may be applicable.[27]

REFERENCES

1. May C, Munro C, Porter M. Alan Lyell (1917-2007) and toxic epidermal necrolysis. J Am Acad Dermatol 60(Suppl 1):AB31, 2009.

2. Bastuji-Garin S, Rzany B, Stern RS, et al. Clinical classification of cases of toxic epidermal necrolysis, Stevens-Johnson syndrome, and erythema multiforme. Arch Dermatol 129:92-96, 1993.

3. Schwartz RA, McDonough PH, Lee BW. Toxic epidermal necrolysis: part I. Introduction, history, classification, clinical features, systemic manifestations, etiology, and immunopathogenesis. J Am Acad Dermatol 69:173,e1-e13, 2013.

4. Farthing P, Bagan JV, Scully C. Mucosal disease series. Number IV. Erythema multiforme. Oral Dis 11:261-267, 2005.

5. Tomasini C, Derlino F, Quaglino P, et al. From erythema multiforme to toxic epidermal necrolysis. Same spectrum or different diseases? G Ital Dermatol Venereol 149:243-261, 2014.

6. Schwartz RA, McDonough PH, Lee BW. Toxic epidermal necrolysis: part II. Prognosis, sequelae, diagnosis, differential diagnosis, prevention, and treatment. J Am Acad Dermatol 69:187,e1-e16, 2013.

7. Kelemem JJ III, Cioffi WG, McManus WF, et al. Burn center care for patients with toxic epidermal necrolysis. J Am Coll Surg 180:273-278, 1995.

8. Abe R. Immunological response in Stevens-Johnson syndrome and toxic epidermal necrolysis. J Dermatol 42:42-48, 2015.

9. Chung WH, Chang WC, Lee YS, et al; Taiwan Severe Cutaneous Adverse Reaction Consortium; Japan Pharmacogenomics Data Science Consortium. Genetic variants associated with phenytoin-related severe cutaneous adverse reactions. JAMA 312:525-534, 2014.

10. Morales ME, Purdue GF, Verity SM, et al. Ophthalmic manifestations of Stevens-Johnson Syndrome and toxic epidermal necrolysis and relation to SCORTEN. Am J Ophthalmol 150:505-510, 2010.

11. Harr T, French LE. Toxic epidermal necrolysis and Stevens-Johnson syndrome. Orphanet J Rare Dis 5:39, 2010.

12. Revuz J, Penson D, Roujeau JC, et al. Toxic epidermal necrolysis: clinical findings and prognostic factors in 87 patients. Arch Dermatol 123:1156-1158, 1987.

13. Auquier-Dunant A, Mockenhaupt M, Naldi L, et al. Correlations between clinical patterns and causes of erythema multiforme majus, Stevens-Johnson syndrome, and toxic epidermal necrolysis: results of an international prospective study. Arch Dermatol 138:1019-1024, 2002.

14. Conway DG, Lyon RF, Heiner JD. A desquamating rash; staphylococcal scalded skin syndrome. Ann Emerg Med 61:118,129, 2013.

15. Mockenhaupt M, Idzko M, Grosber M, et al. Epidemiology of staphylo-coccal scalded skin syndrome in Germany. J Invest Dermatol 124:700-703, 2005.

16. Halebian PH, Corder VJ, Madden MR, et al. Improved burn center survival of patients with toxic epidermal necrolysis managed without corticosteroids. Ann Surg 204:503-512, 1986.

17. Taylor JA, Globe B, Heinbach GM, et al. Toxic epidermal necrolysis. A comprehensive approach. Multidisciplinary management in a burn center. Clin Pediatr 28:404-407, 1989.

18. Sheridan RL, Greenhalgh D. Special problems in burns. Surg Clin North Am 94:781-791, 2014.

19. Heng JS, Malik N, Joshi N, et al. Severity of acute ocular involvement is independently associated with time to resolution of ocular disease in toxic epidermal necrolysis patients. Br J Ophthalmol 99:251-254, 2015.

20. Ducic I, Shalom A, Rising W, et al. Outcome of patients with toxic epidermal necrolysis syndrome revisited. Plast Reconstr Surg 110:768-773, 2002.

21. Heimbach DM, Engrav LH, Marvin JA, et al. Toxic epidermal necrolysis: a step forward in treatment. JAMA 257:2171-2175, 1987.

22. Sheridan RL, Schulz JT, Ryan CM, et al. Long-term consequences of toxic epidermal necrolysis in children. Pediatrics 109:74-78, 2002.

23. Spies M, Sanford AP, Aili Low JF, et al. Treatment of extensive toxic epidermal necrolysis in children. Pediatrics 108:1162-1168, 2001.

24. Mittmann N, Chan B, Knowles S, et al. Intravenous immunoglobulin use in patients with toxic epidermal necrolysis and Stevens-Johnson syndrome. Am J Clin Dermatol 7:359-368, 2006.

25. Chen J, Wang B, Zeng Y, et al. High-dose intravenous immunoglobulins in the treatment of Stevens-Johnson syndrome and toxic epidermal necrolysis in Chinese patients: a retrospective study of 82 cases. Eur J Dermatol 20:743-747, 2010.

26. Barron SJ, Del Vecchio MT, Aronoff SC. Intravenous immunoglobulin in the treatment of Stevens-Johnson syndrome and toxic epidermal necrolysis: a meta-analysis with meta-regression of observational studies. Int J Dermatol 54:108-115, 2015.

27. Kirchhof MG, Miliszewski MA, Sikora S, et al. Retrospective review of Stevens-Johnson syndrome/toxic epidermal necrolysis treatment compar-ing intravenous immunoglobulin with cyclosporine. J Am Acad Dermatol 71:941-947, 2015.

10 Electrical Burns

KEY POINTS

- Electrical injuries can be devastating.
- Many electrical burns damage tissues under the skin.
- Associated injuries must be ruled out.
- Ventricular arrhythmias are common in patients with electrical burns.
- Many patients have long-term effects from electrical injury.

Electrical burns are a unique mechanism of traumatic injury. The extent of damage is usually associated with the voltage, the type of current, the resistance of the tissue, and the duration of contact. Electrical burns account for 5% to 10% of burn unit admissions but are responsible for a disproportionate amount of morbidity and mortality.[1-3] The number of accidents and deaths related to electricity is declining.[4] The main causes of injury include misuse of electrical appliances, inattentiveness, lack of education in safety precautions, and lack of parental supervision.[5] Approximately 81% are occupation-related injuries.[3] Electrical burns occur most frequently in men, then in children, then in women.[6]

PATHOPHYSIOLOGY

Electrical energy is converted to heat, causing thermal injury. Heat generation depends on the strength of the current, the duration of flow, and the resistance of the tissue. Heat is increased when any of those three factors is elevated. Of all tissues, bone has the highest resistance to current but is less damaged by heat. Nerves and vessels generate less heat but are easily damaged (see Chapter 2 for zones of injury). Between the entrance and exit points, the current flows in an unpredictable manner. If the skin resistance is high, less current flows through the body. If low resistance is encountered, such as with sweat or when the person is standing in water, more current will flow through the body. Protein is denatured by electrical current, leading to cell death. Blood vessels are occluded, resulting in anoxia and tissue death. Plasma is lost into the damaged tissue.[7] Major causes of death in electrical burn victims are multiple organ failure and infection.[8]

Electrical burns are categorized into two types: high voltage and low voltage. High-voltage burns (1000 volts or more) usually create more soft tissue damage and are more complex. In addition to the electrical injury, entrance and exit burns occur. With high-voltage burns, thermal burn wounds are possible from the flash of electricity and ignition of clothing.[9]

Lightning can be a unique mechanism of electrical injury. Lightning strike injuries can vary widely, even among groups of people struck at the same time.[10] Lightning can travel underground and exit to patients standing against a metal item. In some victims symptoms are mild and require little medical attention, whereas fatal injuries occur in others.[11,12] Eardrums need to be examined as entrance points. Lightning acts as a direct current shock, as opposed to standard household AC current.[13,14]

Cardiac abnormalities are another common complication of high-voltage injury. The most common cause of death at the scene is ventricular fibrillation. Myocardial infarction can be a direct result of the injury but carries little risk of reinfarction or hemodynamic consequences. The following patient conditions require cardiac monitoring[15]:

- Cardiac arrest
- Cardiac arrhythmias
- 12-lead ECG abnormalities other than bradycardia and tachycardia
- Loss of consciousness
- Severity of burn and patient age, necessitating monitoring

TREATMENT

The burn percentage is used as a guide for fluid resuscitation (see Chapter 3). Additional fluid will be necessary if muscle damage is present. If the urine appears clear, the minimum acceptable rate of production is 0.5 ml/kg/hr. A Foley catheter should be placed to facilitate appropriate monitoring of urine output. If myoglobin or hemoglobin discoloration is noted, increased urine output is needed to prevent renal failure. A guaiac card can be used as a bedside check for myoglobinuria. The treatment of myoglobinuria includes mannitol 0.5 mg/kg IV, followed by 1 ampule of bicarbonate IV. Intravenous fluids are increased until the urine is clear. Mannitol and bicarbonate can be repeated as needed if the urine does not clear or if continuing myoglobinuria is suspected. When bicarbonate is given, the urine should be checked to ensure it is alkaline. If the urine is not alkaline, another ampule of bicarbonate is added to the IV fluids. The bicarbonate is given to prevent precipitation of myoglobin. Precipitated myoglobin and its breakdown products damage the kidney and can lead to renal failure. Acute renal failure occurs in 14.5% of patients. The mortality for patients with renal failure is 59%.[5,16]

AMPUTATION

A high-voltage burn injury frequently necessitates amputation. Deep tissue damage is usually out of proportion to the skin damage. Compartment syndrome is also common. Limbs must be frequently checked for swelling and the 6 Ps: paresthesias, paralysis, pulselessness, poikilothermia, pain, and pallor. Pain out of proportion to passive stretch is a sensitive and specific test. Pallor and pulselessness are late signs. With any suspicion of this syndrome, testing of compartment pressures is essential. Fasciotomies are the preferred modality of treatment. One third of amputees require stump revision because of heterotopic ossification.

The base needs to be well prepared before an amputation site is grafted or closed in patients with electrical injuries, because such injuries often lead to delayed cell death. What looks to be a healthy base during debridement may become necrotic in a couple of days. Serial debridements may be necessary.

LATE SEQUELAE

The sequelae of high-voltage burns often occur in subsequent years. Cataracts develop in 5% to 20% of high-voltage burn patients; they may be amenable to surgery and rehabilitation of sight.[17] Gastrointestinal symptoms include hyperactivity, presenting as vague abdominal complaints and diarrhea. The incidence of biliary disease is increased.

Neurologic syndromes may appear early or late. In most patients the motor system is affected, presenting as a spastic rather than a flaccid syndrome. Weakness is a common clinical finding; this can occur in half of electrical-injury patients.[18] Significant long-term neurologic deficits can persist in 73% of patients (mean follow-up 4½ years). Only 5.3% of patients with a high-voltage burn are able to return to their preinjury occupation.[1] Therefore close, long-term follow-up is critical. Neurologic and psychological symptoms are the most common sequelae of electrical and lightning injuries.[19]

CONCOMITANT INJURIES

Finally, high-voltage electrical burns usually take place when the individual is at a height (e.g., from contact with high-tension lines).

Patients who fall during contact with high voltage must be treated as blunt-trauma victims. All trauma must be evaluated as if the patient was not burned. In patients with electrical injuries, a full-spine radiographic series should be performed to rule out spinal fractures.

Patients with low-voltage injury can usually be treated conservatively, without hospitalization. These are usually household injuries. The exceptions are severe hand burns and large oral injuries that threaten the airway. For these injuries, Neosporin ointment is applied twice a day. It is applied on the lips but not inside the mouth, and if needed, a stretching appliance is used to help restore length and function to the mouth.

Alternating current presents an increased risk of injury because of its tetanic effect. The patient is unable to let go or break contact with the electrical source and thus receives further damage from contact. This tetanic contraction of paravertebral muscles, as well as a fall, can result in axial spine fractures.

REFERENCES

1. Hussmann J, Kincan JO, Russell RC, et al. Electrical injuries—morbidity, outcome, and treatment rationale. Burns 21:530-535, 1995.
2. Xiao J, Cai BR. A clinical study of electrical injuries. Burns 20:340-346, 1994.
3. Brandt MM, McReynolds MC, Ahrns KS, et al. Burn centers should be involved in prevention of occupational electrical injuries. J Burn Care Rehabil 23:132-134, 2002.
4. VanDenburg S, McCormik GM II, Young DB. Investigation of deaths related to electrical injury. South Med J 89:869-872, 1996.
5. Haberal MA. An eleven-year survey of electrical burn injuries. J Burn Care Rehabil 16:43-48, 1995.
6. Lengyel P, Frišman E, Babík J, et al. Electrical burns in our workplace. Acta Chir Plast 56(1-2):13-14, 2014.
7. Fish R. Electric shock. Part I. Physics and pathophysiology. J Emerg Med 11:309-312, 1993.
8. Saracoglu A, Kuzucuoglu T, Yakupoglu S, et al. Prognostic factors in electrical burns: a review of 101 patients. Burns 40:702-707, 2014.
9. Fish R. Electric shock. Part II. Nature and mechanisms of injury. J Emerg Med 11:457-462, 1993.

10. Fahmy FS, Brinsden MD, Smith J, et al. Lightning: the multisystem group injuries. J Trauma 46:937-940, 1999.
11. Patten BM. Lightning and electrical injuries. Neurol Clin 10:1047-1058, 1992.
12. Browne BJ, Gaasch WR. Electrical injuries and lightning. Emerg Med Clin North Am 10:211-229, 1992.
13. Cooper MA. Emergent care of lightning and electrical injuries. Semin Neurol 15:268-278, 1995.
14. American Heart Association. 2005 American Heart Association guidelines for cardiopulmonary resuscitation and emergency cardiovascular care. Part 10.9: Electrical shock and lightning strikes. Circulation 112:IV-154–IV-155, 2005.
15. Hunt JL, Sato R, Baxter C. Acute electric burns. Current diagnostic and therapeutic approaches to management. Arch Surg 115:434-438, 1980.
16. Bittner EA, Shank E, Woodson L, et al. Acute and perioperative care of the burn-injured patient. Anesthesiology 122:448-464, 2015.
17. Chaudhuri Z, Pandey PK, Bhatia A. Electrical cataract: a case study. Ophthalmic Surg Lasers 33:166-168, 2002.
18. Haberal MA, Gurer S, Akman N, et al. Persistent peripheral nerve patholo-gies in patients with electrical burns. J Burn Care Rehabil 17:147-179, 1996.
19. Sanford A, Gamelli RL. Lightning and thermal injuries. Handb Clin Neurol 120:981-986, 2014.

11 Chemical Burns

Chemical burns can occur when a toxic substance is ingested or by direct contact with the skin. Toxic ingestion is commonly seen in adults and adolescents who attempt suicide and in toddlers who ingest toxins accidentally. Burns to the skin are often seen in industrial workers but may also occur through contact with such common household items as alkaline batteries.

INGESTION OF CAUSTICS

The classification of burns of the esophagus is similar to that of burns of the skin. First-degree burns involve the mucosa, with hyperemia, edema, and sloughing. Second-degree burns are transmural.

Third-degree burns erode through the esophagus and involve the periesophageal tissue.

Ingestion of detergents and bleach typically causes only mild esophageal irritation that usually heals without significant morbidity. Acid burns usually cause a coagulation necrosis, which limits their extent. Alkalis produce *liquefaction necrosis*, in which fat and proteins are saponified and blood vessels thrombose. This leads to further cell death. These factors cause alkalis to penetrate deeply and become resistant to surface irrigation.

Solid alkali substances adhere to the mucosal surfaces and rarely reach the stomach in large enough quantities to neutralize acid. Therefore the burns are typically in the oropharynx and mouth and are usually distributed in streaks. The mucosa shows areas of white to dark gray pseudomembranes. The burn produces excessive salivation. A liquid alkali burns all mucosal surfaces. The caustic is usually swallowed, limiting damage to the mouth and pharynx. The major burns are usually to the esophagus and stomach. Reflux pyloric spasm results in the pooling of the alkali in the stomach. Liquid-ingestion burn patients may have odynophagia, dysphagia, and aspiration. They may have retrosternal, back, and peritoneal pain, suggesting mediastinitis or perforation with peritonitis.

TREATMENT

Initially the airway should be surveyed. Intubation may be necessary in patients with laryngospasm, edema, or destruction. Intravenous fluid replacement is started. Broad-spectrum antibiotics are given in patients with an esophageal injury. Steroidal medications have not been shown to be effective. Because they can mask signs of sepsis and peritonitis, we do not use them in our unit.

An upper GI radiographic series will demonstrate damaged mucosa, dilation, and perforation. Gastrografin may be used, although dilute barium will better demonstrate lesions and dilation.

The injury is graded with esophagogastroduodenoscopy (EGD) after the patient is admitted. A small-caliber pediatric scope will minimize injury. The scope can be advanced carefully beyond the known burn to locate a possibly more severe portion not yet detected.

Patients with first-degree burns can be observed for 24 to 48 hours. The rate of stricture formation in these cases is low. Second- and third-degree burns require close attention. Full-thickness necrosis necessitates excision. Restoration of alimentary continuity should be delayed until the patient has recovered from the acute insult. Second- and third-degree burns typically involve esophageal stricture. Dilation is the mainstay of treatment and should be completed 6 to 8 weeks after injury to minimize perforation. Undilatable strictures require esophageal replacement. Percutaneous endoscopic gastrostomy (PEG) tubes may be helpful with dilation procedures. However, if the esophagus is severely injured, a jejunostomy tube can preserve the stomach for a possible esophageal replacement.

CUTANEOUS CHEMICAL BURNS

Chemicals react with the skin, causing damage from oxidation, reduction, desiccation, and corrosion. Destruction usually occurs with a necrotic central zone surrounded by a peripheral hyperemic zone. In most cases lavage with water is the most effective immediate therapy, because it washes away the chemical and dilutes the concentration; exceptions are noted in the following discussion.[1-5]

Alkalis

Alkalis act by dissolving and denaturing proteins. Water is drawn out of the cell, and fat undergoes saponification. They also can cause a protein structure to collapse.

TREATMENT The wound is rinsed with tap water for at least 30 minutes. Ocular injuries should be irrigated with saline solution through a Morgan Lens. Topical ophthalmic anesthetics relieve pain and can stop blepharospasm, which will sometimes interfere with copious irrigation of the eye.[6,7]

Phenols

Phenols are characterized by the substitution of hydrochloral groups for hydrogen groups on a benzene ring. They are found in disinfectants and solvents. They cause skin irritation and can be absorbed cutaneously or inhaled into the lungs. When absorbed, phenols bind to albumin. This can lead to cardiovascular problems (metabolic acidosis, hypertension, and ventricular dysrhythmias), CNS toxicity (coma and seizures), and liver failure. Ingestion of as little as 1 g can be fatal; approximately 50% of all reported cases have a fatal outcome. Only a few patients with high serum concentrations have survived after phenol burns.[8] Phenol is not soluble in water. It is excreted in the urine over a 24-hour period.[9]

TREATMENT   Copious amounts of pure water are used,[10] followed by topical application of surgical sponges soaked with polyethylene glycol. The patient's respiratory and circulatory systems must be stabilized with IV fluid, bicarbonate infusion, and cardiac monitoring. Charcoal should be used for ingestion of a phenol. No antidotes are known, and recovery usually occurs in 1 or 2 days.

Gasoline

An injury from gasoline immersion resembles a small burn. Erythema and blistering are caused by the gasoline's fat-solvent properties. Gasoline contact may cause significant full-thickness burn injuries. Systemic complications can result from the absorption of hydrocarbons through the skin. Regional neuromuscular absorption may produce transient or even permanent impairment.[11] The primary injury caused by gasoline absorption is pulmonary, including bronchitis, pneumonitis, and pneumonic hemorrhages. Gasoline absorbed into the body is excreted by the pulmonary system.[12]

TREATMENT   Skin burns should be cleansed and dressed. Gasoline burns tend to be superficial and heal spontaneously. No antidote is known.[13,14]

Calcium Oxide

Lime burns are common among concrete workers. When cement is dry it contains calcium oxide, which is not particularly dangerous. Calcium oxide and water (often in the form of sweat) react to form calcium hydroxide (an exothermic reaction). Calcium hydroxide is also extremely alkaline (pH 12 to 13); normal human skin has a pH of 5.5. The initial burn under clothing often is not painful; a victim may not know until hours later that he or she has been burned. The burns are often deep and appear to be "punched out" of the skin.[15]

TREATMENT   Lime residue should be brushed away before the skin is washed. Contaminated clothing is removed. The area is copiously irrigated with water until it no longer feels soapy. The patient is then dried thoroughly.

Hydrofluoric Acid

Hydrofluoric acid is used in glassware etching. It is also found in some bleach and cleaning agents. It can cause life-threatening hypocalcemia and hypomagnesemia. Patients with hypocalcemia from this cause usually do not show the typical signs. Hydrofluoric acid–induced hypocalcemia is identified through serum calcium levels and ECG findings.[16] It can cause ventricular fibrillation that is particularly resistant to treatment.[17]

TREATMENT   The injury is treated with immediate application of 2.5% calcium chloride ointment (usually while the patient is being transported). This is followed by injection of 10% calcium gluconate into the subcutaneous tissues. Digital block is usually performed after areas of pain are marked. When the block wears off, reinjection is necessary if pain persists. Even if the block is not complete, it is a briefly painful procedure, and the pain will cease when all of the hydrofluoric acid is neutralized. Some injuries involve a large surface area such as the entire hand, as seen with gloves soaked with the acid. Treatment consists of placement of a brachial arterial line, followed by 4 to 6 hours of infusion of 10 ml of 10% calcium gluconate in 50 ml of normal saline solution, until the pain is relieved. This is repeated as needed until pain is relieved. Multiple infusions are usually necessary.[18]

New treatments may be on the horizon. Hexafluorine has been shown to be effective for cutaneous and eye splash exposure to hydrofluorane.[19-21]

Significant exposures require cardiac monitoring, IV access, and initial and continuing monitoring of electrolytes, including calcium, magnesium, and potassium. Patients are monitored for ECG changes such as QT prolongation and evidence of hypocalcemia. Intravenous infusion of bicarbonate will enhance renal excretion of fluoride. Hemodialysis may become necessary.[17,22]

Phosphorus

Phosphorus melts at body temperature and invades deep into the body tissue. Phosphorus burns are painful. Care should be taken when copper sulfate is used as an antidote, because copper toxicity can present a danger; the copper will be excreted renally. Hypocalcemia and hyperphosphatemia can occur, with associated myocardial arrhythmias and sudden death.

TREATMENT The patient's clothes must be removed immediately, because they may ignite or reignite. During transportation of the patient, the wound should be covered with a saline- or water-soaked dressing. On arrival, the wound is continuously irrigated with saline solution or water. Phosphorus is washed out of the wound, which is submerged in a tub of saline solution or water. Alternatively, phosphorus is directly removed using a dilute copper sulfate solution

(0.5%), which deactivates the phosphorus and turns it black to facilitate removal.

Adequate urinary output (0.5 ml/kg/hr) must be maintained by giving fluids or diuretics. The ECG should be monitored and serial measurements of calcium and phosphate levels obtained.[23-26]

REFERENCES

1. Pruitt VM. Work-related burns. Clin Occup Environ Med 5:423-433, 2006.
2. Tan T, Wong DS. Chemical burns revisited: what is the most appropriate method of decontamination? Burns 41:761-763, 2015.
3. Brent J. Water-based solutions are the best decontaminating fluids for dermal corrosive exposures: a mini review. Clin Toxicol (Phila) 51:731-736, 2013.
4. Tovar R, Leikin JB. Irritants and corrosives. Emerg Med Clin North Am 33:117-131, 2015.
5. Dinis-Oliveira RJ, Carvalho F, Moreira R, et al. Clinical and forensic signs related to chemical burns: a mechanistic approach. Burns 41:658-679, 2015.
6. Lorette JJ, Wilkinson JA. Alkaline chemical burn to the face requiring full thickness skin grafting. Ann Emerg Med 17:739-741, 1988.
7. Bunker DJ, George RJ, Kleinschmidt A, et al. Alkali-related ocular burns: a case series and review. J Burn Care Res 35:261-268, 2014.
8. Horch R, Spilker G, Stark GB. Phenol burns and intoxications. Burns 20:45-50, 1994.
9. Vearrier D, Jacobs D, Greenberg MI. Phenol toxicity following cutaneous exposure to Creolin®: a case report. J Med Toxicol 11:227-231, 2015.
10. Abbate D, Polito I, Puglisi A, et al. Dermatosis from resorcinol in tire makers. Br J Ind Med 46:212-214, 1989.
11. Schneider MS, Mani MM, Masters FW. Gasoline-induced contact burns. J Burn Care Rehabil 12:140-143, 1991.
12. Kim HK, Takematsu M, Biary R, et al. Epidemic gasoline exposures following Hurricane Sandy. Prehosp Disaster Med 28:586-591, 2013.
13. Hunter GA. Chemical burns of the skin after contact with petrol. Br J Plast Surg 21:337-341, 1968.
14. Walsh WA, Scarba FJ, Brown RS, et al. Gasoline immersion burn. N Engl J Med 291:830-833, 1974.

15. Chung JY, Kowal-Vern A, Latenser BA, et al. Cement-related injuries: review of a series, the National Burn Repository, and the prevailing literature. J Burn Care Res 28:827-834, 2007.
16. Mayer TG, Gross PL. Fatal systemic fluorosis due to hydrofloric acid burns. Ann Emerg Med 14:149-153, 1985.
17. McIvor ME, Cummings CE, Mower MM, et al. Sudden cardiac death from acute fluoride intoxication: the role of potassium. Ann Emerg Med 16:777-781, 1987.
18. Robinson EP, Chhabra AB. Hand chemical burns. J Hand Surg Am 40:605-612, 2015.
19. Mathieu L, Nehles J, Blomet J, et al. Efficacy of hexafluorine for emergent decontamination of hydrofluoric acid eye and skin splashes. Vet Hum Toxicol 43:263-265, 2001.
20. Sheridan RL, Ryan CM, Quinby WC Jr, et al. Emergency management of major hydrofluoric acid exposures. Burns 21:62-64, 1995.
21. Yoshimura CA, Mathieu L, Hall AH, et al. Seventy per cent hydrofluoric acid burns: delayed decontamination with Hexafluorine® and treatment with calcium gluconate. J Burn Care Res 32:e149-e154, 2011.
22. Robinett DA, Shelton B, Dyer KS. Special considerations in hazardous materials burns. J Emerg Med 39:544-553, 2010.
23. Davis KG. Acute management of white phosphorus burn. Mil Med 167:83-84, 2002.
24. Barqouni L, Abu Shaaban N, Elessi K. Interventions for treating phosphorus burns. Cochrane Database Syst Rev 6:CD008805, 2014.
25. Al Barqouni LN, Skaik SI, Shaban NR, et al. White phosphorus burn. Lancet 376:68, 2010.
26. Barillo DJ, Cancio LC, Goodwin CW. Treatment of white phosphorus and other chemical burn injuries at one burn center over a 51-year period. Burns 30:448-452, 2004.

12 Pediatric Burn Management

KEY POINTS

- Children have thin skin; therefore their injuries tend to be deep, complicated by contracture and hypertrophic scarring.

- Children have a higher metabolic rate than that calculated using standard equations for adults.

- Early excision and coverage has become more accepted in the treatment of pediatric burns.

- Burned children should be hospitalized if abuse is the suspected cause, and the incident must be reported to authorities.

- Children often desire less reconstruction than that recommended by their surgeons.

INCIDENCE/EPIDEMIOLOGY

In the United States, 136,453 children were injured from a fire or burn and treated in emergency rooms in 2012. This number includes more than 67,000 children 4 years of age and younger.[1,2]

In 2011, 325 children 19 years of age or younger died from fires or burns, 277 (85%) of which occurred in residential fires; 47% of children who died from fires or burns were 4 years of age or younger. The death rate for children this age (0.77 per 100,000) is almost twice that of 5 to 9 year olds (0.40 per 100,000) and almost four times that of 10 to 14 year olds (0.20 per 100,000). The death rate from fires and burns decreased by 55% from 1999 to 2011.[1,2]

Young children, especially those 5 years of age or younger, are at the greatest risk from home fire-related death and injury. The fire death rate for this age group is twice the national average. These children have a less-acute perception of danger, less control over their environment, and a limited ability to react promptly and properly to a fire.[3]

Every day more than 300 children 19 years of age or younger are treated in emergency departments for burn-related injuries, and two of these children die. Younger children are more likely to have scald burns caused by hot liquids or steam, whereas older children are more likely to be burned by direct contact with fire.[4]

Fire and burn injuries are the second leading cause of death in children. (The first is general trauma.) Survival rates have improved in this population. The current management of pediatric burn injuries has led to at least a 50% chance of survival in patients with an otherwise uncomplicated 90% to 95% burn injury.[5,6] The mortality rate increases significantly with smoke inhalation injury. Almost 70% of deaths in children are from inhalation of smoke and/or toxic gases; thermal injury is responsible for 30%.[3]

The overall improvement in mortality and outcome can be attributed to many factors, including early and aggressive resuscitation, respiratory care and treatment of inhalation injury, control of infection, early burn excision and grafting, and treatment of the hypermetabolic response to trauma.[7] Higher-volume burn centers have been shown to improve outcomes.[8]

MONETARY IMPACT

The total annual cost of fire- and burn-related deaths among children 14 years of age or younger is more than $2.6 billion. The cost for those 4 years of age or younger is more than $1.4 billion.[3,9,10]

Every dollar spent on a smoke alarm can save $69 in fire-related deaths.[9]

UNIQUE PATIENT POPULATION

Pediatric patients are not just little adults—this is a unique patient population with unique challenges and responses. A child's skin is thinner than an adult's skin; thus it provides less protection from thermal injury. The same heat exposure causes a more severe burn injury in a child than in an adult. Children's injuries are likely to be deeper and to be complicated by contracture and hypertrophic scarring. Secondary disfigurement often exceeds the damage of the original burn wound.[11-13]

RESUSCITATION

Key issues in pediatric trauma include the following:
- Airway
- Access
- Ambient temperature

As with adults, pediatric patients are trauma patients and should be treated as such. Advanced trauma life support protocols need to be applied.

Airway

Inhalation injury, with the attendant infection and pulmonary failure, is a primary determinant of mortality in thermally injured children. It is definitively diagnosed by bronchoscopy. The smaller opening of a pediatric airway predisposes it to obstruction. A 1 mm increase in tissue thickness of a 4 mm diameter pediatric trachea results in a 16-fold increase in resistance and a 75% reduction of the cross-sectional area. In an adult, the same increase in tissue thickness would increase the airway resistance only threefold and reduce the airway area by 44%.[14]

Hyperextension of the neck is contraindicated in pediatric patients. Direct laryngoscopy is necessary to examine the larynx and cords for soot or edema. A straight blade is used in children less than 6 years of age. A rule of thumb is to use an endotracheal tube the diameter of the child's unburned small finger. We typically use an uncuffed endotracheal tube.

A tracheostomy may be performed in pediatric patients to secure the airway after admission. The duration of a tracheostomy depends on the extent of the burn.[15]

Access

Children with large burn injuries may require two large-vessel access points. Central-vein canalization can be difficult. Femoral or saphenous veins may be the best routes for large-vein access, with a surgical cutdown if necessary. If needed, intraosseous access can be obtained.

Hypovolemic shock can present quickly in pediatric burn patients. This is especially true of infants, because their losses are proportionately larger. For example, 20% TBSA in a child weighing 10 kg causes an evaporative loss of 475 ml, or 60% of the circulating volume. The same burn in an adult weighing 70 kg would result in a loss of 1.1 L, or only 20% of the patient's circulating volume.

Ambient Temperature

Infants and toddlers are prone to hypothermia because of their increased surface-to-volume ratio, decreased insulating fat, and lower muscle mass (for shivering). Caregivers should attempt to reduce heat loss. The ambient temperature should be 28° to 32° C (82° to 90° F). Bathing and/or showering should be done quickly, without unnecessary exposure.

Surface Area Calculations

Burn wounds are most accurately mapped after loose tissue, soot, and dirt are washed off. Children have a larger surface area per unit weight. Infants have a larger surface area of the head, with less surface area on the extremities, compared with adults. Thus the *rule of nines* must be modified to calculate the TBSA in pediatric patients (see Fig. 3-2, p. 20).

In a child younger than 1 year of age, the head is approximately 19% of the body mass, and the extremities account for 13% each. A useful rule for calculating this percentage is the following: For each year older than 1, 1% is subtracted from the head, and 0.5% is added to each lower extremity. A useful rule for estimating burn size is the following: The palmar surface of a child's hand is approximately 1%. This can be used clinically for nonuniform areas.

The Berkow table and the Lund/Browder body chart (see Fig. 3-3, p. 21) are the most accurate resources for TBSA and should be used for definitive documentation and calculation.[16]

Resuscitation Formulas: Modified Parkland

The Parkland formula is modified in pediatric patients by adding maintenance fluid to the resuscitation fluid volume as follows (Table 12-1):

$$(4 \text{ ml LR} \times \text{kg} \times \%\text{TBSA}) + (\text{Maintenance fluid}) =$$
$$\text{Amount to be given in the first 24 hours}$$

For example, the maintenance fluid requirement for a 30 kg patient is calculated as follows:

$$100 \times 10 \text{ (for the first 10 kg)} + 50 \times 10 \text{ (for the second 10 kg)} +$$
$$20 \times 10 \text{ (for the 10 kg not yet covered)}:$$
$$1000 + 500 + 200 = 1700 \text{ ml/24 hr} = 70 \text{ ml/hr}$$

Table 12-1 Method for Calculating Maintenance Fluid

First 10 kg	100 ml/kg
Second 10 kg	50 ml/kg
Every kilogram above 20 kg	20 ml/kg

Half of the total fluid is given in the first 8 hours after the burn injury; the other half is given in the next 16 hours. The fluid of choice is lactated Ringer's (LR) solution. Infants may require glucose if the blood level on a finger-stick sample is less than 80 mg/dl. For these patients, D5LR is given. In the first 8 hours of resuscitation, we add 1 ampule of bicarbonate for each liter of LR for increased sodium needs. In the third 8-hour period after the burn, we add 1 ampule of salt-poor albumin (SPA) to each liter of LR.

These are starting points; the rate should be individualized for each patient. The desired urine output is 1 ml/kg/hr. Because of decreased urine-concentrating abilities in infants, placement of a Foley catheter is essential to monitor output.[17]

During the second 24 hours, 0.45% NaCl is given as replacement because of the small intravascular volume of children; 5% dextrose is added. If only D5W is given and the infusion rate is too rapid, hyponatremia and seizure may result.[18] Our fluid of choice is D5½NS. The fluid rate is titrated to urine output and perfusion status.

We try to increase the hourly rate and avoid bolus. When needed, fluid boluses of normal saline (NS) solution are given in amounts of no more than 25% of the total circulating volume: Total body volume = 10 ml/kg of body weight.

Electrolytes should be monitored for hyponatremia and hypokalemia. (Supplementation may be needed). Losses should be replaced as potassium phosphate, not potassium chloride, because hypophosphatemia is frequently observed. If hypokalemia is present, the magnesium level should be evaluated. Care is required to prevent volume overload.[19]

PEDIATRIC BURN PHYSIOLOGY

A child's heart is less compliant than an adult's, and stroke volumes plateau at relatively low filling pressures. This shifts the Starling curve to the left. Cardiac output (CO) depends almost exclusively on heart rate, and an immature heart is more sensitive to volume and pressure overload.

Children are prone to the development of edema. They require particular monitoring for cerebral edema. The head needs to be elevated, especially in the first 24 to 48 hours after a burn injury. Frequent neurologic assessments are needed. Pulmonary edema is often caused by hydrostatic pressures, and in the absence of an inhalation injury, is almost diagnostic of fluid overload. Treatment of overhydration includes fluid restriction and diuresis.

Blood loss should be replaced on the second day after a burn injury. The usual amount of blood replacement in a 24-hour period is 10 ml/kg, infused over 3 to 4 hours. Unless active blood loss is observed, no more than 15 ml/kg should be given over any 24-hour period. Larger quantities can result in cardiopulmonary congestion or severe hypertension.

Adequacy of Resuscitation

The usual signs of hypovolemia in an adult (tachycardia, hypotension, and decreased urine output) are late signs in a pediatric patient. Children have remarkable cardiopulmonary reserve. They often do not show signs of hypovolemia until more than 25% of their circulating volume is lost, when cardiovascular collapse is imminent. This population frequently develops reflex tachycardia secondary to catecholamine release, even with minimal to moderate stress levels. A smaller body size allows lower vascular pressures to circulate the blood. Therefore systolic pressures of less than 100 mm Hg are common in children 5 years of age or younger.

Young children with immature kidneys have less tubular concentrating ability. Urine production may continue despite the presence of hypovolemia.

More reliable indicators include mental clarity, pulse pressures, arterial blood gases, distal extremity color and warmth, capillary refill, and body temperature. If more than three of these indicators are abnormal, the child is in danger. Table 12-2 summarizes normal pediatric vital signs; Table 12-3 contrasts adult and pediatric Glasgow Coma Scale indicators.

Table 12-2 Normal Pediatric Vital Signs

Age (years)	Heart Rate (beats/min)	Systolic Blood Pressure (mm Hg)	Respirations (breaths/min)
<2	100-160	60	30-40
2-5	80-140	70	20-30
6-12	70-120	80	18-25
>12	60-110	90	16-20

Table 12-3 Glasgow Coma Scale

Adults		Infants/Toddlers	
Eye Opening (E)			
Spontaneous	4	Spontaneous	4
To speech	3	To speech	3
To pressure	2	To pain	2
None	1	None	1
Verbal Response (V)			
Oriented	5	Coos, babbles	5
Confused	4	Irritable, cries	4
Words	3	Cries to pain	3
Sounds	2	Moans to pain	2
None	1	None	1
Motor Response (M)			
Obeying commands	6	Spontaneous moves	6
Localising	5	Withdraws to touch	5
Normal flexion (withdrawal)	4	Withdraws to pain	4
Abnormal flexion	3	Abnormal flexion	3
Extension	2	Abnormal extension	2
None	1	None	1

Adult scale from Teasdale G, Maas A, Lecky F, et al. The Glasgow Coma Scale at 40 years: standing the test of time. Lancet Neurology 13:844-854, 2014. Pediatric scale from Kirkham FJ, Newton CR, Whitehouse W. Paediatric coma scales. Dev Med Child Neurol 50:267-274, 2008.

Metabolism/Nutrition

Children younger than 3 years of age, especially infants younger than 6 months, have a limited amount of glycogen stored in their liver. This may rapidly deplete during times of stress. Initiation of protein and lipid catabolism for gluconeogenesis is accelerated. Thus blood glucose should be measured every hour for the first 24 hours after a burn injury to prevent hypoglycemia.

Children are growing, and their metabolic rates are higher than those predicted by adult equations. Major catastrophic illnesses and trauma can produce transient and permanent changes in growth. In severe burns, growth of nails, hair, and bone may be slowed and usually do not catch up after injury. Children often will refuse to eat anything, much less enough calories for basic energy expenditure and healing. This is most often true in children with a TBSA of more than 20%. NOTE: **Do *not* confuse BSA (body surface area) with TBSA (total *burned* surface area).**

Galveston Formula

Infants	2100 kcal/m^2 BSA $+ 1000 \text{ kcal/m}^2$ TBSA
Toddlers	2100 kcal/m^2 BSA $+ 1000 \text{ kcal/m}^2$ TBSA
School-age children	1800 kcal/m^2 BSA $+ 1300 \text{ kcal/m}^2$ TBSA
Adolescents	1500 kcal/m^2 BSA $+ 1500 \text{ kcal/m}^2$ TBSA

Body Surface Area Equation

$$[87(H + W) - 2600] \div 10,000 = \text{Surface in m}^2$$

where H equals the height in centimeters and W equals the weight in kilograms. (The TBSA is computed using the diagrams on Fig. 3-2 on p. 20.)

Modified Curreri Formula

Infants	BMR + (15 kcal $\div$ %TBSA)
Toddlers	BMR + (25 kcal $\div$ %TBSA)
School-age children	BMR + (40 kcal $\div$ %TBSA)
Adolescents	BMR + (40 kcal $\div$ %TBSA)

Basal Metabolic Rate Equation

Male =
66.5 + (13.7 × Weight in kg) + (5 × Height in cm) − (6.8 Age)
Female =
65.5 + (9.6 × Weight in kg) + (1.7 × Height in cm) − (4.7 Age)

Children will tolerate enteral feedings through a gastric or duodenal tube 3 to 6 hours after a burn injury. Hyperosmolar feeds should not be given, because they can cause diarrhea. Caregivers should work with anesthesia colleagues to minimize the length of preoperative NPO orders.

WOUND CARE: RECONSTRUCTION, TIMING, AND OTHER ISSUES

The goal of burn wound care is to preserve function and provide the best cosmetic result. Topical antimicrobials should be secured with thick, fluffy dressings. Surginet (expandable fishnet) dressings and splints may be helpful. Children should be observed to ensure that they do not eat the topical creams. At least once a day, wounds are bathed, inspected for infection, and redressed.

Early excision and grafting can be undertaken.[20,21] Decisions are made on an individual case basis by those with experience and expertise in the management of these wounds. The management of pediatric burns has changed over the years to one of early excision and coverage. The benefits of this approach include less time in the hospital and fewer episodes of infection.[20,22] Surgeons should consider repeated scar release and the application of skin grafts during the patient's growth-spurt years.[23] Occasionally, negative pressure dressings are useful.[24]

Rehabilitation is a key element, is started early, and continues throughout the long-term follow-up. When joints are not exercised, they should be splinted in extension. The hands and neck are most prone to contracture.[25,26]

Although some patients surviving severe burns have lingering disability, most have a satisfying quality of life. Comprehensive burn care that includes experienced, multidisciplinary aftercare is essential in the recovery process.[21]

Scald Injuries

Scalds are common in children.[12,27] Burns to the neck, shoulder, and thoracic wall in young children are almost always caused by scalding with hot liquids. Adequate release of neck contractures is essential because of the risk of impaired growth and micrognathia.[28] Anterior chest scald injuries usually produce deep second- or third-degree burns. The mammary gland is not usually affected. The mammary gland is an epithelial gland and receives its blood supply from posterior to the gland. The burn is typically superficial and not one of breast volume. Treatment is conservative, with release of the soft tissue envelope at puberty to allow future breast development, and later resurfacing with a skin graft or flap, as needed.

Electrical Cord Bites

Electrical cord bites are the most common electrical injury in children; 90% of these injuries occur in children younger than 4 years of age. The boy/girl incidence is 2:1. This is not a conductive heat injury. Tissue destruction can be extensive. No immediate reconstruction is attempted.

Splinting the oral commissure with orthodontic appliances is the recommended treatment; the appliances are worn for 9 to 12 months. Delayed reconstruction can be performed, if necessary. This treatment modality requires a cooperative patient and parents and frequent monitoring by a prosthodontist. Roughly a fourth of patients have bleeding from the labial artery, typically 1 to 2 weeks after the injury. Parents should be instructed to apply pressure for several minutes when this occurs.[29]

Excision of the burn scar with restoration of the labial muscula-ture can be attempted to reduce the number of contractions postop-eratively.[30-32] Ventral tongue flaps have also been applied.[33]

Some will debride and perform definitive repair in the first 2 weeks after a burn injury. This approach is usually not recommend-ed unless the combined loss of commissure and lower lip exceeds a third of the length of the lip.[34]

Toxic Epidermal Necrolysis Syndrome

Toxic epidermal necrolysis syndrome (TENS) is an acute inflammatory systemic disease that results in extensive epidermal sloughing (see Chapter 9). The burn unit is the appropriate place for management of these patients because of the need for intensive monitoring, dress-ing changes, and physical/occupational therapy. Intubation is neces-sary if the airway is involved. Prevention of wound desiccation and infection is essential for these patients' survival and functional recov-ery. Biologic dressings are used. Enteral feedings are started early. Steroid medications are not given. Antibiotics are given to manage specific foci of infection only.[35-37] The SCORTEN scale and other predictive models may help to predict morbidity and mortality.[38,39]

UNIQUE ISSUE IN CHILDREN: ABUSE

Often, a burn or scald injury in a child is evidence of neglect or abuse. This may account for 20% of pediatric burn admissions.[40] Most of these injuries are scald or contact burns in children younger than 3 years of age. The Child Abuse Prevention and Treatment Act of 1974 requires professionals to report suspected abuse. Caregivers should not hesitate to admit these patients to the hospital if a dan-gerous home situation is a possible cause.

Signs Suggesting Abuse

- The child is brought for treatment by an unrelated adult.
- There is an unexplained delay of 12 hours in seeking treatment.
- Parental affect is inappropriate: inattentive to the child, lacking empathy, possibly under the influence of alcohol or drugs.
- A sibling of the patient is blamed for the injury.
- The injury is inconsistent with the description of the circumstances of the injury.
- The injury is inconsistent with the developmental capacity of the patient.
- The prior history includes accidental or nonaccidental injury to the patient or siblings.
- The prior history includes failure to thrive.
- Historical accounts of the injury differ with each interview.
- The injury is localized to the perineum, genitalia, and/or buttocks.
- Mirror-image injuries are present on the extremities.
- The child's affect is inappropriate (withdrawn and flat).
- The child shows evidence of unrelated injuries (e.g., bruises, scars, welts, and fractures).

PSYCHOSOCIAL CONSIDERATIONS

A patient's priorities for reconstruction may differ from those of his or her parents and the surgeons. In one study, patients usually desired less reconstruction than parents, especially older children.[41] Adolescents desired cosmetic (as opposed to functional) reconstruction. Most of the severely burned patients wanted only one procedure. These patients had accepted their appearance more readily than those with less severe burns.

Psychological support is important to ensure the best outcome. Numerous social support groups exist in the local community, nationally, and on the Internet. Family and friends are essential in supporting the patient's long-term treatment and rehabilitation—but they, too, may need support in coping with the experience.[42]

SAMPLE ADMISSION ORDERS

(Do not write comments—shown here in italics—on the order sheet.)

ADMISSION

To pediatric burn unit

DX

s/p trauma, 30% TBSA burn secondary to house fire

HEIGHT AND WEIGHT

CONDITION

Critical

VITAL SIGNS

Per routine. [Continuous monitoring of vitals. Record qh; call HO if temp >39° C (102.5° F), P <60 or >100, BP <110 systolic or >160 systolic, pulse ox <90. Strict I&O qh; notify HO if <1.0 ml/kg/hr]. Monitor CVP, record qh.

ALLERGIES

(Document allergies and monitor drug interactions.)

ACTIVITY

Bed rest. Head of bed at a 20-degree angle *(to minimize cerebral and tracheal edema)*. No pillow for head and neck burns *(to minimize contractures and damage to ears)*.

NURSING

Per routine. Wound care as per unit protocol. *(See Chapter 5 for examples of such a protocol.)*

DIET

NPO if burn >30%. Enteral feedings with TraumaCal or a similar formula. *(Target feedings of 25 kcal/kg/day × 2.0 [stress factor].) (See pp. 160-161 to determine caloric need [goal].)*
Tube feedings:

½ strength @ 25 ml/hr × 4 hr, then
¾ strength @ 25 ml/hr × 4 hr, then
Full strength @ 25 ml/hr × 4 hr, then
Increase 15 ml/q4h to goal.
Check residuals q4h; hold if >150 ml.

IV FLUIDS

The Parkland formula is modified in pediatric patients by adding maintenance fluid to the resuscitation fluid volume.

$$(4 \text{ ml LR} \times \text{kg} \times \%\text{TBSA}) + (\text{Maintenance fluid}) =$$
$$\text{Amount to be given in first 24-hr period}$$

Resuscitation fluid: (4 ml LR × kg × %TBSA)
Give half in the first 8-hr period.
Give half in the next 16-hr period.

In addition to the resuscitation fluid, the maintenance fluid is given at a steady rate over the first 24 hours (see Table 12-1). The fluid of choice is LR solution. Infants may require glucose. In the first 8 hours of resuscitation, we add 1 ampule of bicarbonate for each liter of LR solution for increased sodium needs. In the third 8-hour burn period after the burn injury, we add 1 ampule of SPA.

NOTE: SPA is a 25% solution. Therefore the calculation is 0.1 ml × kg × %TBSA. If the institution uses only Plasmanate (a 5% colloid solution), the calculation for colloid administration is 0.5 ml × kg × %TBSA.

EXAMPLE: Start IV LR at ___ ml/hr for ___ hours. Add 1 amp $NaCO_2$ to IV fluids. (If glucose level from a finger-stick sample is <80 mg/dl, start D5LR). Then decrease LR to ___ml/hr for 16 hours. Give 1 unit SPA in each liter of LR, starting 16 hours after the burn. During the second 24 hours, D/C LR (or D5LR). Start ½ NS at current rate. Adjust fluid rate titrated to urine output (1.0 ml/kg/hr). Follow finger stick to determine whether D5 should be added.

MEDICATIONS

Topical Antibiotics

Silver sulfadiazine (Silvadene) on body; bacitracin-polymyxin B (Polysporin) on face

Mycostatin (Nystatin) 200,000 U PO/NGT q8h *(to inhibit bacterial transorption)*

Tetanus toxoid 0.5 ml IM

Hypertet 250 U IM *(for patients whose history of immunization is not available)*

Carafate 1 g PO/NGT q6h *(if >20% burn)*

MVI 10 ml IV qd

Pain Medications

Dilaudid 2 mg IV q4h

MSO_4 8 mg IV q4h

Other Agents

Heparin 2500 U (weight dependent) SQ q8h

Codeine 30 mg PO q6h prn *(altered physiology, hyperosmolar fluids cause diarrhea)*

ADDITIONAL ORDERS

If the patient has an eye burn:

Polysporin ophthalmic solution *(Double-check that the Polysporin solution and/or ointment is the ophthalmic type.)*

If the patient has a pulmonary injury:

Aminophylline 6.0 mg/kg IV load, then 0.5 mg/kg/hr IV

Ventolin 0.5 mg in 2 ml NS via nebulizer q4h and prn

Heparin 4000 U (mix with Ventolin nebulizer in the 2 ml NS) will help to decrease pulmonary casts

(Consider bronchoscopic evaluation.)

If the patient has no pulmonary injury:

Oxygen per nasal cannula or high-humidity face mask

Chest physical therapy

If the patient has an electrical injury:

Complete spine series *(Be sure to visualize C7-T1.)*

Long-bone radiographic film series

Urine myoglobin and hemoglobin assay

EXTRA ORDERS

NGT to LCWS flush q2h with 30 ml NS

Daily weight measurement

Bed in 20-degree semi-Fowler position

Elevate extremities

Foot cradle, splints

Abduct shoulders

Foley to gravity

Decubitus precautions

No pillow for a head/neck burn

VENTILATOR SETTINGS AND PEEP

Preferred ventilator: VDR_4

Initial settings

Oscillatory rate 600 cycles per minute

PIP 30-35 cm H_2O
2 sec inspiration
2 sec expiration

If your institution does not have this equipment available, use the following standard ventilator settings. For nonburn patients, usually start on AC 10, VT of 10-15 ml/kg, 100% FIO_2, PEEP 5 cm H_2O. Burn patients require increased respiratory rate and decreased tidal volume, because contraction from the burn limits chest expansion. Therefore start at AC 15-20, VT 6 ml/kg. Check an ABG in 30 min and make adjustments accordingly.

Obtain an ABG 30 min after the patient is placed on the ventilator *(and make changes accordingly).*

ABG/carboxyhemoglobin *(on admission and prn)*

ECG *(on admission and prn)*

CXR *(on admission. We usually obtain one on M, F, and prn. A CXR is obtained qd for intubated patients. Assess for infiltrate, tube placement, pneumothorax.)*

LABORATORY TESTS

CBC *(on admission and W)*

SMA-12 *(on admission and M)*

SMA-7 *(on admission, M-W-F, and prn)*

PT/PTT *(on admission and prn)*

Sputum C&S *(on admission and prn)*

Ca, Mg, Phos *(on admission and biweekly)*

H&H/electrolytes *(q8h until the patient is stable, and then prn)*

Finger-stick blood sugar *(on admission and q4h and prn)*

Urine 24-hr electrolytes *(on admission)*

HIV/EtOH/urine drug screen *(on admission)*

B-hCG *(if patient is female)*

Sickle cell panel *(if patient is black)*

Eschar BX *(prn)*
Albumin, prealbumin, transferrin *(qw [on M])*

CONSULTATIONS

OT/PT
Nutrition

OTHER CONSULTATIONS *(prn)*

(Consent is required for HIV testing, placing central lines, grafting, blood transfusions.)

REFERENCES

1. Centers for Disease Control and Prevention, National Center for Injury Prevention and Control. Web-based Injury Statistics Query and Reporting System (WISQARS). Unintentional fire/burn fatalities and injuries, children ages 19 and under. Available at *http://www.cdc.gov/injury/wisqars/index.html.*
2. Safe Kids Worldwide. Burns and fire safety fact sheet, 2014.
3. Safe Kids Worldwide. Facts about injuries to children by residential fires, 2004.
4. Centers for Disease Control and Prevention, National Center for Injury Prevention and Control. Protect the ones you love: child injuries are preventable. Available at *http://www.cdc.gov/safechild/.*
5. Sheridan RL, Remensnyder JP, Schnitzer JJ, et al. Current expectations for survival in pediatric burns. Arch Pediatr Adolesc Med 14:245-249, 2000.
6. Kraft R, Herndon DN, Al-Mousawi AM, et al. Burn size and survival probability in paediatric patients in modern burn care: a prospective observational cohort study. Lancet 379:1013-1021, 2012.
7. Herndon DN, Spies M. Modern burn care. Semin Pediatr Surg 10:28-31, 2001.
8. Palmieri TL, Taylor S, Lawless M, et al. Burn center volume makes a difference for burned children. Pediatr Crit Care Med 16:319-324, 2015.
9. Injury facts, burn injury. National Safe Kids Campaign, 2002. Children's National Medical Center. Available at www.*SafeKids.org.*
10. Hill D. Personal communication. Landover, MD: Children's Safety Network, Economics and Insurance Resource Center, 2004.
11. Harmel RP Jr, Vane DW, King DR. Burn care in children: special considerations. Clin Plast Surg 13:95-105, 1986.

12. Trop M, Herzog SA, Pfurtscheller K, et al. The past 25 years of pediatric burn treatment in Graz and important lessons been learned. An overview. Burns 41:714-720, 2015.

13. Gonzalez R, Shanti CM. Overview of current pediatric burn care. Semin Pediatr Surg 24:47-49, 2015.

14. Breitman M. Burn physiology. Scritti Biol 7:395-398, 1932.

15. Sen S, Heather J, Palmieri T, et al. Tracheostomy in pediatric burn patients. Burns 41:248-251, 2015.

16. Goverman J, Bittner EA, Friedstat JS, et al. Discrepancy in initial pediatric burn estimates and its impact on fluid resuscitation. J Burn Care Res 2014 Nov 18. [Epub ahead of print]

17. Merrell S, Saffle JR, Sullivan JJ, et al. Fluid resuscitation in thermally injured children. Am J Surg 152:664-669, 1986.

18. O'Neil CE, Hutsler D, Hildreth MA. Basic nutritional guidelines for pediatric burn patients. J Burn Care Rehabil 10:278-284, 1989.

19. Deitch EA, Rutan RL. The challenges of children: the first 48 hours. J Burn Care Rehabil 21:424-430, 2000.

20. Xiao-Wu W, Herndon DN, Spies M, et al. Effects of delayed wound excision and grafting in severely burned children. Arch Surg 137:1049-1054, 2002.

21. Sheridan RL, Hinson MI, Liang MH, et al. Long-term outcome of children surviving massive burns. JAMA 283:69-73, 2000.

22. Hunt JL, Purdue GF, Pownell PH, et al. Burns: acute burns, burn surgery and postburn reconstruction. Sel Read Plast Surg 8:1-37, 1997.

23. Goldberg DP, Kucan JO, Bash D. Reconstruction of the burned foot. Clin Plast Surg 27:145-161, 2000.

24. Koehler S, Jinbo A, Johnson S, et al. Negative pressure dressing assisted healing in pediatric burn patients. J Pediatr Surg 49:1142-1145, 2014.

25. Atiyeh B, Janom HH. Physical rehabilitation of pediatric burns. Ann Burns Fire Disasters 27:37-43, 2014.

26. Luce JC, Mix J, Mathews K, et al. Inpatient rehabilitation experience of children with burn injuries: a 10-yr review of the Uniform Data System for Medical Rehabilitation. Am J Phys Med Rehabil 94:436-443, 2015.

27. Shah A, Suresh S, Thomas R, et al. Epidemiology and profile of pediatric burns in a large referral center. Clin Pediatr (Phila) 50:391-395, 2011.

28. Almaguer E, Dillon BT, Parry SW. Facial resurfacing at Shriners Burns Institute: a 16-year experience in young burned patients. J Trauma 25:1081-1082, 1985.

29. Yeroshalmi F, Sidoti EJ Jr, Adamo AK, et al. Oral electrical burns in children—a model of multidisciplinary care. J Burn Care Res 32:e25-e30, 2011.

30. Pensler JM, Rosenthal AM. Reconstruction of the oral commissure after an electrical burn. J Burn Care Rehabil 11:50-53, 1990.

31. Silverglade D, Ruberg RL. Nonsurgical management of burns to the lips and commissures. Clin Plast Surg 13:87-94, 1986.
32. Leake JE, Curtin JW. Electrical burns of the mouth in children. Clin Plast Surg 11:669-683, 1984.
33. Donelan MB. Reconstruction of electrical burns of the oral commissure with a ventral tongue flap. Plast Reconstr Surg 95:1155-1164, 1995.
34. Ortiz-Monasterio F, Factor R. Early definitive treatment of electrical burns of the mouth. Plast Reconstr Surg 65:169-176, 1980.
35. Sheridan RL, Weber JM, Schulz JT, et al. Management of severe toxic epidermal necrolysis in children. J Burn Care Rehabil 20:497-500, 1999.
36. Spies M, Sanford AP, Aili Lao JF, et al. Treatment of extensive toxic epidermal necrolysis in children. Pediatrics 108:1162-1168, 2001.
37. Sheridan RL, Schulz JT, Ryan CM, et al. Long-term consequences of toxic epidermal necrolysis in children. Pediatrics 109:74-78, 2002.
38. Beck A, Quirke KP, Gamelli R, et al. Pediatric toxic epidermal necrolysis: using SCORTEN and predictive models to predict morbidity when a focus on mortality is not enough. J Burn Care Res 36:167-177, 2015.
39. Quirke KP, Beck A, Gamelli RL, et al. A 15-year review of pediatric toxic epidermal necrolysis. J Burn Care Res 36:130-136, 2015.
40. Leetch AN, Woolridge D. Emergency department evaluation of child abuse. Emerg Med Clin North Am 31:853-873, 2013.
41. Bjarnason D, Phillips LG, McCoy B, et al. Reconstructive goals for children with burns: are our goals the same? J Burn Care Rehabil 13:389-390, 1992.
42. Rimmer RB, Bay RC, Alam NB, et al. Measuring the burden of pediatric burn injury for parents and caregivers: informed burn center staff can help to lighten the load. J Burn Care Res 36:421-427, 2015.

Appendix

GLOSSARY

AA	Amino acid
ABG	Arterial blood gas
AC	Assist control
Ant	Anterior
APRV	Airway pressure release ventilation
ARDS	Acute respiratory distress syndrome
BCAA	Branched-chain amino acid
BEE	Basal energy expenditure
B-hCG	Beta-human chorionic gonadotropin
bid	Twice per day *(bis in die)*
BMR	Basal metabolic rate
BP	Blood pressure
BSA	Body surface area (not burned surface area)
BUN	Blood urea nitrogen
BX	Biopsy
C	Compliance
Ca	Calcium
C&S	Culture and sensitivity
CBC	Complete blood cell count
C_{dyn}	Dynamic compliance
CEA	Cultured epithelial autograft
CHO	Carbohydrate
CO	Cardiac output
CO_2	Carbon dioxide

CPAP	Continuous positive airway pressure
Cr	Creatinine
Cstat	Static compliance
CT	Computed tomography
CVP	Central venous pressure
CXR	Chest x-ray
D/C	Discontinue
ΔP	Change in pressure
ΔV	Change in volume
D5½NS	5% Dextrose in 0.45% sodium chloride
D5LR	5% Dextrose in lactated Ringer's solution
D5W	5% Dextrose in water
dl	Deciliter
DX	Diagnosis
ECG	Electrocardiogram
ECMO	Extracorporeal membrane oxygenation
EFA	Essential fatty acid
EGD	Esophagogastroduodenoscopy
EM	Erythema multiforme major
ER	Emergency room
EtOH	Ethanol
ETT	Endotracheal tube
F	Friday
FENa	Fractional excretion of sodium
FFA	Free fatty acid
FIO_2	Fraction of inspired oxygen (how much oxygen is dialed into ventilator to have the patient breathe)
FRC	Functional residual capacity
GCS	Glasgow Coma Scale
GI	Gastrointestinal
H&H	Hemoglobin and hematocrit
Hb	Hemoglobin
HCO_3	Bicarbonate

HFV	High-frequency ventilation
HIV	Human immunodeficiency virus
HLA	Human leukocyte antigen
HO	House officer
H$_2$O	Water
hr	Hour
HX	History
I&O	Input and output ("ins and outs")
IBD	Inflammatory bowel disease
IM	Intramuscular
IV	Intravenous
JP	Jackson-Pratt urinary drain
K	Potassium
kg	Kilogram
LCWS	Low continuous wall suction
LFT	Liver function test
LLE	Left lower extremity
LR	Lactated Ringer's (solution)
LUE	Left upper extremity
M	Monday
MCT	Medium-chain triglyceride
mg	Milligram
Mg	Magnesium
MgSO$_4$	Magnesium sulfate
min	Minute
ml	Milliliter
µg	Microgram
MVI	Multivitamin infusion
MVO$_2$	Mixed venous oxygen saturation
MVP	Moisture vapor permeable (film)
M-W-F	Monday-Wednesday-Friday
N	Sodium
Na	Sodium

NaCl	Sodium chloride
NGT	Nasogastric tube
NO$_2$	Nitrous oxide (mnemonic: Us = 2, like 2 oxygens)
NO$_3$	Nitric oxide
NPO	Nothing by mouth *(nil per os)*
NS	Normal saline (solution)
O$_2$	Oxygen
OR	Operating room
OT	Occupational therapy
P	Pulse
PACO$_2$	Partial pressure of carbon dioxide in the alveoli
PaCO$_2$	Partial pressure of carbon dioxide in the blood
PAO$_2$	Partial pressure of oxygen in the alveoli
PaO$_2$	Partial pressure of oxygen in the blood
PAP	Pulmonary artery pressure
PCO$_2$	Partial pressure (arterial air pressure) of carbon dioxide
PCV	Pressure-control ventilation
PEEP	Positive end-expiratory pressure
PEG	Percutaneous endoscopic gastrostomy
pH	Acidity-alkalinity measure
Phos	Phosphorus
PIP	Peak inspiratory pressure
PO	By mouth *(per os)*
PO$_2$	Partial pressure of oxygen
POD	Postoperative day #____
Post	Posterior
PRBC	Packed red blood cell
prn	As needed *(pro re nata)*
PT	Prothrombin time, physical therapy
PTT	Partial thromboplastin time
qd	Once every day *(quoque die)*
qh	Every hour *(quaque hora)*

q4h	Every 4 hours
q6h	Every 6 hours
q12h	Every 12 hours
qid	Four times per day *(quater in die)*
qw	Every week
RDA	Recommended dietary allowance
RLE	Right lower extremity
RR	Respiratory rate
RUE	Right upper extremity
SCORTEN	Score of Toxic Epidermal Necrosis
SIMV	Synchronized intermittent mandatory ventilation
SJS	Stevens-Johnson syndrome
SMA-7, SMA-12	Sequential Multiple Analyzer blood chemistry tests
s/p	Status post
SPA	Salt-poor albumin
SQ	Subcutaneously
STSG	Split-thickness skin graft
SSSS	Staphylococcal scalded skin syndrome
SVO$_2$	Mixed venous oxygen saturation *(See also MVO$_2$)*
SVR	Systemic vascular resistance
TBSA	Total burned surface area
tbsp	Tablespoon
TENS	Toxic epidermal necrolysis syndrome
tid	Three times per day *(ter in die)*
Tmax	Maximum temperature per a given time period (usually 24 hours)
TNF-a	Tumor necrosis factor–alpha
TNL	Total nitrogen loss
2,3-DPG	2,3Diphosphoglycerate
TPN	Total parenteral nutrition
TX	Treatment; therapy
U	Units

UO	Urine output
UUN	Urinary urea nitrogen
V/Q	Ventilation/perfusion
VT	Tidal volume
W	Wednesday
WBC	White blood cell (count)
ZnSO$_4$	Zinc sulfate

MORITZ CONTACT CHART

A burn is the transfer of heat to tissue. The depth of the injury depends on the intensity of the heat and the duration of the contact to produce a full-thickness burn injury.

Temperature		
°F	°C	**Time for a Third-Degree Burn**
156		1 sec
150	66	2 sec
149		2 sec
140	60	5 sec
133		15 sec
130	54	30 sec
127		60 sec
125	52	2 min
124		3 min
120	49	10 min

From Moritz AR, Henriques FC. Studies of thermal injury: II. The relative importance of time and surface temperature in the causation of cutaneous burns. Am J Pathol 23:695-720, 1947.

USEFUL RANGES AND EQUATIONS

CVP	Central venous pressure	1-8 mm Hg
MAP	Mean arterial pressure	75-100 mm Hg
PCWP	Wedge pressure	5-12 mm Hg
CO	Cardiac output	4-6 L/min
CI	Cardiac index	2-4 L/min/m^2
SVR	Systemic vascular resistance	800-1200 dynes $\times$ sec/cm^5
PVR	Peripheral vascular resistance	100-200 dynes $\times$ sec/cm^5
CaO$_2$	Arteriovenous oxygen content	16-22 ml O$_2$/100 ml
	(SaO$_2$ $\times$ Hb $\times$ 1.39) + PaO$_2$ $\times$ 0.0031)	
CvO$_2$	Venous oxygen content	12-17 ml O$_2$/100 ml
	(SvO$_2$ $\times$ Hb $\times$ 1.39) + (PvO$_2$ $\times$ 0.0031)	
C(a-v)O$_2$	Arteriovenous oxygen difference	3.5-5.5 ml O$_2$/100 ml
	CaO$_2$ $-$ CvO$_2$	
DO$_2$	Oxygen delivery CaO$_2$ $\times$ CO $\times$ 10	700-1400 ml/min
VO$_2$	Oxygen consumption C(a-v)O$_2$ $\times$ CO $\times$ 10	150-300 ml/min
O$_2$ER	Oxygen extraction ratio VO$_2$/DO$_2$	0.23-0.32

Index

A

A-a (alveolar-arterial) gradient equation, 98-100

A-aO$_2$ (alveolar-arterial oxygen) difference (DA-aO$_2$), 98-100

ABG (arterial blood gas) measurements, 92-94

  determination of base deficit from, 94-95

Absorbent foam for wound cleansing, 116

Abuse, child, 163-164

Acid burns from ingestion of caustics, 145

Acinetobacter infection, 55

Activity

  for pediatric patients, 165

  on sample admission orders, 34

Acute hospitalizations for burn injuries, 2

Admission orders

  for pediatric patients, 165-170

  sample, 34-39

Admission to burn unit

  indications for, 48-50

  sample admitting orders for, 34-39

  statistics on, 2

AgNO$_3$ (silver nitrate), 63

Airway

  admission for monitoring of, 50

  constriction and obstruction of, 90

  with pediatric burns, 154-155

  in primary survey, 16

  in secondary survey, 16

Airway pressure release ventilation (APRV), 92

Albumin, salt-poor (SPA)

  for pediatric patients, 157, 166-167

  in resuscitation, 23, 76

  on sample admission orders, 35

Albuterol, inhaled nebulized heparin mixed with, 88

Alkali burns

  cutaneous, 146-147

  from ingestion of caustics, 145

Allergies on sample admission orders, 34

Allied health practitioners, 43-44

Alloderm for wound closure, 59-60

Allograft for wound closure, 59

Alveolar-arterial (A-a) gradient equation, 98-100

Alveolar-arterial oxygen (A-aO$_2$) difference (DA-aO$_2$), 98-100

Ambient temperature for pediatric patients, 155

Amphotericin B, 64

Amputation for electrical burn, 140-141

Antibiotics

  for inhalation injury, 90

  intravenous (IV), 44

  parenteral, 60, 61

  for pediatric patients, 167

  on sample admission orders, 36

  topical, 36, 56, 61-64

  for wound sepsis, 55, 60-64

Antifungal agents for wound sepsis, 64

Antioxidants, 78, 79
APRV (airway pressure release venti-
lation), 92
Arterial blood gas (ABG) measure-
ments, 92-94
determination of base deficit from,
94-95
Asboe-Hansen sign, 131
Ascorbic acid in wound healing, 105
Aspergillus infection, 55
Assessment of other parameters, 24
Autolytic cleansing products, 117

B
Bacterial infection, 55, 60-64
Basal energy expenditure (BEE),
72-73
Basal metabolic rate (BMR), 68-69,
72, 73
Basal metabolic rate (BMR) equation,
161
Base deficit, determination from arte-
rial blood gas of, 94-95
BCAAs (branched-chain amino acids),
70
Bed, choice of, 44, 114-115
Bed rest
for pediatric patients, 165
on sample admission orders, 34
Bedsores; *See* Pressure sores
Berkow's percentages chart, 18, 21, 22
Betadine (povidone-iodine ointment),
62
Beta-hemolytic *Streptococcus* infection,
55, 58
Bicarbonate (HCO_3) replacement,
95-96
Blood loss in pediatric patients, 158
Body diagram, 18-21
Body surface area (BSA), 18, 23

Body surface area (BSA) equation, 160
Braden scale, 109-110
Bradykinin, 9, 10
Branched-chain amino acids (BCAAs),
70
Breathing
in primary survey, 16
in secondary survey, 16-17
Burn(s)
classification of, 6-7
first-degree, 6, 7
pathophysiology of, 5-12
second-degree, 6, 7, 8
third-degree, 6, 7
Burn edema, 9, 10-11, 17
Burn injury(ies)
economic impact of, 2-3
emergency room visits for, 2
epidemiology of, 1
inpatient acute hospitalizations
for, 2
physiologic response to, 9-12
zones of, 7-9
Burn size lethal to 50% of population
(LD_{50}), 54
Burn unit
admission to, 34-39
introduction to, 1-3
Byrd ventilators, 88

C
Cadaver skin for wound coverage, 59
Calcium oxide, cutaneous burns from,
148
Calcium requirements, 77
Caloric needs, 72-74
Candida albicans infection, 55, 58
Candida krusei infection, 55
Candida tropicalis infection, 55

Carbon dioxide (CO_2) laser for scar revision, 51
Carbon dioxide (CO_2) level, ventilator setting and, 96-97
Carbon monoxide poisoning, 86-87
Carboxyhemoglobin levels, 86-87
Cardiac index, 68
Cardiac output in pediatric patients, 157
Caustics, ingestion of, 144-146
CD8+ T cells in toxic epidermal necrolysis syndrome/Stevens-Johnson syndrome, 130-131
Central access, 17
Central venous pressure (CVP) catheters, changing of, 44
Cerebral edema in pediatric patients, 158
Chemical burns, 144-151
    cutaneous, 146-150
        from alkalis, 146-147
        from calcium oxide, 148
        from gasoline, 147-148
        from hydrofluoric acid, 148-149
        from phenols, 147
        from phosphorus, 149-150
    from ingestion of caustics, 144-146
Chemical cleansing products, 118
Chemoattractants in wound healing, 104
Chemotherapy and wound healing, 123
Chest burn, circumferential, 89
Child abuse, 163-164
Children; *See* Pediatric burns
Chloride requirements, 77
Circulation
    in primary survey, 16
    in secondary survey, 17-18
Circumferential chest burn, 89
Classification of burns, 6-7

Cleansing products, 116-118
Clysis, 60
CO_2 (carbon dioxide) laser for scar revision, 51
CO_2 (carbon dioxide) level, ventilator setting and, 96-97
CO_2/O_2 (respiratory quotient), 73-74
Coagulation, zone of, 7, 8
Coagulation system, activation of, 9, 10
Collagen phase of wound healing, 104-105
Collagenase/Polysporin powder, 62
Coma scale, 159
Compartment syndrome from electrical burn, 140-141
Compliance equation, 100
Condition on sample admission orders, 34
Consultations
    for pediatric patients, 170
    on sample admission orders, 39
Contamination of wound, 106
Continuous positive airway pressure (CPAP), 92
Contractures, follow-up care for, 51-52
Corium, 5, 7, 8
Creams for skin protection, 119
Critical care, organization for notes and presentation on, 39-41
Critical care formulas, 81
Crucial formula, 81
Crystalline sodium chloride dressing
    for mechanical cleansing, 118
    for wound cleansing, 117
Curreri formula, modified, 160
Cutaneous chemical burns, 146-150
    from alkalis, 146-147
    from calcium oxide, 148
    from gasoline, 147-148

from hydrofluoric acid, 148-149
from phenols, 147
from phosphorus, 149-150
CVP (central venous pressure) cathe-
    ters, changing of, 44
Cyanide, 90

D

DA-aO$_2$ (A-aO$_2$ difference), 98-100
Debridement, 24, 41, 115
Decontamination of wound, 106
Decubitus ulcers; *See* Pressure sores
Deep second-degree burns, 6, 7, 8
Dermis, 5, 7, 8
Diagnosis on sample admission or-
    ders, 34
Diet
    for pediatric patients, 166
    on sample admission orders, 35
Dietitians, 43-44
Diflucan (fluconazole), 64
Direct excision for full-thickness
    burns, 59
Disability
    in primary survey, 16
    in secondary survey, 18
Discharge to home, 45
Dressings, silver-impregnated, 64
Drug(s), toxic epidermal necrolysis
    syndrome/Stevens-Johnson
    syndrome from, 129-130

E

ECMO (extracorporeal membrane
    oxygenation), 92
Economic impact of burn injuries, 2-3
Ectoderm, 5
Edema
    burn, 9, 10-11, 17
    cerebral, 158
    generalized, 9

interstitial, 9
in pediatric patients, 158
pulmonary, 158
upper airway, 89
Elbows, escharotomy of, 28-29
Elderly patient, sample admission or-
    ders for, 37
Electrical burns, 138-143
    from alternating current, 142
    amputation for, 140-141
    concomitant injuries with, 141-142
    epidemiology of, 138
    high-voltage versus low-voltage,
        139-140, 141-142
    late sequelae of, 141
    from lightning, 139
    pathophysiology of, 139-140
    pediatric, 168
    sample admission orders for, 37
    treatment of, 140
Electrical cord bites, 162-163
Electrolytes
    in pediatric patients, 157
    requirements for, 77
EM (erythema multiforme major) ver-
    sus toxic epidermal necrolysis
    syndrome/Stevens-Johnson
    syndrome, 129, 133
Emergency room visits for burn in-
    juries, 2
Endotracheal intubation, 88
Ensure Plus, 81
Ensure pudding, 81
Enteral feedings
    available formulas for, 78-81
    parenteral versus, 71-72, 78
    for pediatric patients, 166
    on sample admission orders, 35
Enterobacter infection, 55, 58
Enzymes for chemical cleansing, 118
Epidemiology of burn injuries, 1

Epidermis, 5, 7, 8
Epithelial proliferation and migration in wound healing, 105-106
Erythema multiforme major (EM) versus toxic epidermal necrolysis syndrome/Stevens-Johnson syndrome, 129, 133
Eschar as culture medium, 58
Escharectomy, 58
Escharotomy, 24-33
Escherichia coli infection, 55, 58
Evaluation, initial, 14-15
Excisions, repeat, 42
Exposure
    in primary survey, 16
    in secondary survey, 18-21
Extracorporeal membrane oxygenation (ECMO), 92
Extremity burns, 42-43
Extubation, 98
Eye burn
    in pediatric patient, 168
    sample admission orders for, 37

F
Facial burns, 42
Fat, calories from, 73-74
Feet, escharotomy of, 32-33
Fever workup, 44
Fibrinogen in wound healing, 104
Fibroblastic phase of wound healing, 104-105
First-degree burns, 6, 7
Fluconazole (Diflucan), 64
Fluid(s)
    in nutritional support, 76-77
    for pediatric patients, 166-167
Fluid resuscitation, 22-23, 76-77
Foam dressings for skin protection, 119

Foam skin for skin cleansing, 116
Follow-up care, 50-52
Full-thickness burns, initial wound management for, 59-60
Fungal infection, 55, 58, 64

G
Galveston formula, 160
Gasoline, cutaneous burns from, 147-148
Gel(s)
    for wound cleansing, 116
    for wound protection, 120
Gelatin/pectin wafers for wound protection, 120
Generalized edema, 9
Gentamicin, 63
Glasgow Coma Scale, 159
Glucerna, 80
Glutamine, 70
Grafts, skin, 42, 58, 121
    split-thickness, 59
Granulation tissue, 115

H
Hand burns, 42-43
    admission for, 50
    escharotomy of, 27
Harris-Benedict equation, 72-73
HCO_3 (bicarbonate) replacement, 95-96
Health shakes, 81
Heparin, inhaled nebulized, 88
HFV (High-frequency ventilation), 91
High-frequency ventilation (HFV), 91
High-voltage burns, 139-140, 141-142
History-taking, 15
Home, discharge to, 45
Hospitalizations for burn injuries, 2

Hydrocolloids
  for autolytic cleansing, 117
  for wound protection, 120
Hydrofluoric acid, cutaneous burns
       from, 148-149
Hydrogels
  for autolytic cleansing, 117
  for wound cleansing, 116
Hydrophilic-hydrophobic absorbent
       foam for wound cleansing, 116
Hyperemia, zone of, 8, 9
Hyperglycemia, 71
Hypermetabolism, 12, 68-69
Hypertrophic scarring, 51
Hypoproteinemia, 9
Hypothermia
  in pediatric patients, 155
  prevention of, 24
Hypovolemia in pediatric patients,
       158-159
Hypovolemic shock in pediatric pa-
       tients, 155

I
Impregnated gauze
  for mechanical cleansing, 118
  for wound cleansing, 117
Infected wounds, 54-58, 60-64, 122
Inflammation, 9, 10-11
Inflammatory phase of wound heal-
       ing, 104
Inhalation injury, 85-100
  carbon monoxide poisoning from,
       86-87
  diagnosis of, 87-88
  epidemiology of, 85-86
  morality from, 85-86
  pathophysiology of, 89-90
  pediatric, 154-155

  treatment of, 88, 90-100
    A-a gradient equation in, 98-100
    antibiotics for, 90
    bicarbonate replacement in,
       95-96
    Byrd ventilators for, 88
    changing ventilator setting to
       change CO_2 level in, 96-97
    compliance equation in, 100
    determination of base deficit
       from arterial blood gas in,
       94-95
    inhaled nebulized heparin mixed
       with albuterol for, 88
    inhaled nitrous oxide for, 88
    oxygenation for, 88, 91-92, 98
    preparing to extubate in, 98
    pulmonary toilet for, 90
    steroids for, 90-91
    ventilation for, 91-92
    ventilator management in, 92-94
Inhaled nebulized heparin mixed with
       albuterol, 88
Inhaled nitrous oxide, 88
Initial evaluation, 14-15
Initial resuscitation, 15-23
  history-taking in, 15
  primary survey in, 16
  secondary survey in, 16-23
Inpatient acute hospitalizations for
       burn injuries, 2
Integra for wound closure, 59, 60
Interstitial edema, 9
Intravenous (IV) access, 17
Intravenous (IV) antibiotics, 44
Intravenous (IV) fluids on sample ad-
       mission orders, 35
Inverse-rate ventilation, 91
Iron levels, 78
Irrigations for mechanical cleansing,
       118

J
Jevity, 80

K
Keratinocytes in toxic epidermal
    necrolysis syndrome/Stevens-
    Johnson syndrome, 130
Klebsiella infection, 55, 58

L
Laboratory tests
    for pediatric patients, 169
    on sample admission orders, 38-39
Lactated Ringer's (LR) solution,
    22, 76
    for pediatric patients, 157
Lag phase of wound healing, 104
LD_{50} (burn size lethal to 50% of pop-
    ulation), 54
Leg(s), escharotomy of, 30-31
Leg ulcerations, 123-124
Legal action, 15
Leukocytes in wound healing, 104
Lightning, electrical burns from, 139
Lime burns, 148
Lind, James, 105
Lipolysis, 71
Liquefaction necrosis, 145
Liquid skin for skin cleansing, 116
Logrolling, 17-18
Lotions for skin protection, 119
Low tidal volume ventilation, 92
Low-voltage burns, 139, 142
Lower airways, damage to, 89-90
LR (lactated Ringer's) solution, 22, 76
    for pediatric patients, 157
Lyell, Alan, 128
Lyell syndrome, 129

M
Mafenide acetate (Sulfamylon), 63
Magnesium requirements, 77
Maintenance fluids
    for pediatric patients, 156
    in resuscitation, 22-23, 76-77
    on sample admission orders, 35
Marjolin, Jean-Nicolas, 106
Marjolin's ulcer, 106
Maturation phase of wound healing,
    105
MCT (medium chain triglycerides)
    oil, 81
Mechanical cleansing products, 118
Mechanism of injury, 15
Medications on sample admission
    orders, 36
Medium chain triglycerides (MCT)
    oil, 81
Mesoderm, 5
Metabolism
    effects of injury on, 69
    in pediatric patients, 160-161
Methicillin-resistant *Staphylococcus au-
    reus* (MRSA) infection, 55, 58
Miconazole, 64
Minute ventilation, 94, 96
Moisture vapor permeable (MVP)
    film
    for autolytic cleansing, 117
    for skin protection, 119
MRSA (Methicillin-resistant
    Staphylococcus aureus) infection,
    55, 58
Muscle wasting, 69-71
MVP (Moisture vapor permeable)
    film
    for autolytic cleansing, 117
    for skin protection, 119

Myocutaneous flaps, 121, 122
Myoglobinuria from electrical burns,
    140

N
Na (sodium)
    requirements for, 77
    serum, 23
NaCl (sodium chloride) for pediatric
    patients, 157
Nasogastric tube (NGT), 72
Nasotracheal intubation, 88
Necrotic tissue, excision of, 58
Negative pressure wound therapy
    (NPWT), 115-120
Nepro, 80
Newborn, skin surface area of, 5
NGT (Nasogastric tube), 72
Nikolsky sign, 131
Nitrogen balance, 75
Nitrous oxide, inhaled, 88
Normal saline for wound cleansing,
    117
Norton scale, 108-109
NPO
    for pediatric patients, 166
    on sample admission orders, 35
NPWT (Negative pressure wound
    therapy), 115-120
Nursing per routine
    for pediatric patients, 166
    on sample admission orders, 35
NutriHep, 80
Nutrition, 68-84
    enteral versus parenteral, 71-72,
        78-82
    injury, metabolic rate, and stress
        factors for, 69-71
    nutritional support for, 71-78
    in pediatric patients, 160-161

Nutritional support, 71-78
    antioxidants in, 78, 79
    caloric and protein needs in, 72-75
    electrolytes in, 77
    enteral versus parenteral, 71-72,
        78-82
    fluids in, 76-77
    for toxic epidermal necrolysis syn-
        drome/Stevens-Johnson syn-
        drome, 135
    trace elements in, 78
    vitamins in, 77
Nystatin, 64

O
Occupational therapists, 43
Ointments
    for skin protection, 119
    for wound protection, 120
Oral modifiers, 81
Oral supplements, 81
Orotracheal intubation, 88
Outpatient care, 50-52
Oxygen consumption, 68
Oxygen saturation, 92-93
Oxygen-hemoglobin dissociation
    curve, 93
Oxygenation, 88, 91-92
    evaluation of, 98
    extracorporeal membrane, 92
    management of, 92-94

P
Pain management
    admission for, 50
    outpatient care for, 51
    for pediatric patients, 167
    on sample admission orders, 36
Palliative care, 52
Palmar surface, 18

Parenteral antibiotics, 60, 61
Parenteral feedings
    complications of, 78, 79
    enteral versus, 71-72, 78
Parkland formula
    for pediatric patients, 156-157,
        166-167
    for resuscitation, 22, 76
    on sample admission orders, 35
Partial-thickness burns, initial wound
        management for, 58
Past medical history, 15
Pasteur, Louis, 58
Pathogens, 57-58
Pathophysiology of burns, 5-12
PCO_2, 94, 96-97
PCV (pressure-control ventilation),
        91, 92
Pectin wafers for wound protection,
        120
Pediatric burns, 152-172
    from abuse, 163-164
    incidence/epidemiology of, 152-
        153
    monetary impact of, 153-154
    physiology of, 157-161
        and adequacy of resuscitation,
            158-159
        metabolism/nutrition in, 160-
            161
    psychosocial considerations with,
        164-165
    resuscitation for, 154-157
        access in, 155
        adequacy of, 158-159
        airway in, 154-155
        ambient temperature in, 155
        resuscitation formulas (modified
            Parkland) for, 156-157
        surface area calculations in, 155-
            156

    rule of nines for estimating total
        burned surface area in, 20
    sample admission orders for, 165-
        170
    as unique population, 154
    wound care for, 161-163
        for electrical cord bites, 162-163
        for scald injuries, 162
        for toxic epidermal necrolysis
            syndrome, 163
PEEP (positive end-expiratory pres-
        sure)
    for inhalation injury, 91-92
    for pediatric patients, 168-169
    on sample admission orders, 38
PEG (percutaneous endoscopic gas-
        trostomy) tube, 72
Peptamen, 81
Perative, 81
Percutaneous endoscopic gastrostomy
        (PEG) tube, 72
Peripheral vascular disease, leg ulcer-
        ations from, 124
Phenols, cutaneous burns from, 147
Phosphate requirements, 77
Phosphorus, cutaneous burns from,
        149-150
Physical therapists, 43
Physiologic response to burn injury,
        9-12
Pigskin for wound coverage, 59
Plasmanate on sample admission or-
        ders, 36
Pneumonia, 86, 89, 148
PO_2, 92-93
Positive end-expiratory pressure
        (PEEP)
    for inhalation injury, 91-92
    for pediatric patients, 168-169
    on sample admission orders, 38
Posttraumatic stress, 52

Potassium requirements, 77
Povidone-iodine ointment (Betadine), 62
Preoperative evaluation, 41
Pressure garments for hypertrophic scarring, 51
Pressure reduction/relief devices, 114-115
Pressure sores, 107-121
    assessment of
        Braden scale for, 109-110
        Norton scale for, 108-109
    classification of, 110-111
    prognosis for, 121
    risk factors for, 107-108
    treatment of, 111-121
        debridement for, 115
        negative pressure wound therapy for, 115-120
        pathway to design new system for, 111, 112-113
        pressure reduction/relief devices for, 114-115
        principles for, 111
        surgical coverage for, 121
        wound care products for, 115, 116-120
        wound care team for, 111
Pressure-control ventilation (PCV), 91, 92
Primary survey, 16
ProMod, 81
Protection products, 119-120
Protein catabolism, 69-70
Protein needs, 74-75
Protein nutritional status, assessment of, 75
Proteus infection, 55, 58
Providentia infection, 55, 58
Pseudomonas aeruginosa infection, 55, 58

Pseudomonas infection, 55
Psychiatric care, 45
Psychosocial considerations for pediatric patients, 164-165
Pulmocare, 80
Pulmonary edema in pediatric patients, 158
Pulmonary injury
    in pediatric patient, 168
    sample admission orders for, 37
Pulmonary toilet, 90

R
Radiotherapy and wound healing, 122-123
Rehabilitation, 45
    for pediatric patients, 161
Remodeling phase of wound healing, 105
Resource formula, 81
Respiratory embarrassment from circumferential chest burn, 89
Respiratory quotient (CO_2/O_2), 73-74
Resuscitation
    initial, 15-23
    for pediatric burns, 154-157
        access in, 155
        adequacy of, 158-159
        airway in, 154-155
        ambient temperature in, 155
        resuscitation formulas (modified Parkland) for, 156-157
        surface area calculations in, 155-156
    in secondary survey, 22-23
Resuscitation formulas, for pediatric patients, 156-157
Ringer's solution, lactated, 22, 76
    for pediatric patients, 157

Ritter disease versus toxic epidermal
  necrolysis syndrome/Stevens-
  Johnson syndrome, 133-134
Rule of nines, 19, 20, 22
  for pediatric patients, 156

S
Salt-poor albumin (SPA)
  for pediatric patients, 157, 166-167
  in resuscitation, 23, 76
  on sample admission orders, 35
Scald injuries, pediatric, 162
Scarring, 51
SCORe of Toxic Epidermal Necrolysis
  (SCORTEN) scale, 132-133
Secondary survey, 16-23
  airway in, 16
  breathing in, 16-17
  circulation in, 17-18
  disability in, 18
  exposure in, 18-21
  resuscitation in, 22-23
Second-degree burns, 6, 7, 8
Semiocclusive foam dressings for skin
  protection, 119
Semiocclusive moisture vapor perme-
  able (MVP) film
  for autolytic cleansing, 117
  for skin protection, 119
Sepsis, 54-58, 60-64
Sequential eschar excision for
  full-thickness burns, 59
Serotonin, 9, 10
Serratia infection, 55, 58
Serum Na, 23
Silicone for hypertrophic scarring, 51
Silver nitrate (AgNO$_3$), 63
Silver sulfadiazine (Silvadene), 62
Silver-impregnated dressings, 64
SJS; *See* Stevens-Johnson syndrome

Skeletal muscle, 70
Skin
  anatomy of, 5
  functions of, 5
Skin cleansing products, 116
Skin grafts, 42, 58, 121
  split-thickness, 59
Skin protection products, 119
Skin sealants for skin protection, 119
Skin surface area, 5
Skin thickness, 5
Sodium (Na)
  requirements for, 77
  serum, 23
Sodium chloride (NaCl) for pediatric
  patients, 157
SPA (salt-poor albumin)
  for pediatric patients, 157, 166-167
  in resuscitation, 23, 76
  on sample admission orders, 35
Specialty formulas, 80
Split-thickness skin grafts, 59
Sprays for skin protection, 119
SSSS (staphylococcal scalded skin
  syndrome, versus toxic epi-
  dermal necrolysis syndrome/
  Stevens-Johnson syndrome),
  133-134
Staged excision for full-thickness
  burns, 59
Standard formulas, 80
Staphylococcal scalded skin syndrome
  (SSSS) versus toxic epidermal
  necrolysis syndrome/Stevens-
  Johnson syndrome, 133-134
Staphylococcus aureus, methicillin-resis-
  tant, 55, 58
Staphylococcus infection, 55, 57-58
Stasis, zone of, 8, 9
Step-down burn care, 44-45
Steroids for inhalation injury, 90-91

Stevens-Johnson syndrome (SJS),
        128-137
    causes of, 129-130
    clinical presentation of, 131-132
    defined, 129
    differential diagnosis of, 129, 133-
        134
    epidemiology of, 129
    historical background of, 128-129
    pathophysiology of, 130-131
    prognosis for, 132-133
    treatment of, 134-135
Streptococcus infection, 55
Stress factors, 69-70, 73
Subcutaneous fat, 7
Subcutaneous tissue, 8
Substrate phase of wound healing, 104
Sugar free health shakes, 81
Sulfamylon (mafenide acetate), 63
Superficial second-degree burns, 6,
        7, 8
Suplena, 80
Surface area calculations, 19, 20, 22
    for pediatric patients, 155-156
Surgical coverage of wounds, 121
Survey
    primary, 16
    secondary, 16-23

T

TBSA (Total burned surface area), 9,
        18-21
    pediatric, 160-161
Temporary wound coverage, 59
TENS; *See* Toxic epidermal necroly-
        sis syndrome
Tetanus prophylaxis, 61
Third-degree burns, 6, 7
Thrombosis, 9, 10
Tidal volume (V_T), 91
TNL (total nitrogen loss), 75

Topical antibiotics
    for pediatric patients, 167
    on sample admission orders, 36
    for wound care, 56, 61-64
Total burned surface area (TBSA), 9,
        18-21
    pediatric, 160-161
Total nitrogen loss (TNL), 75
Total parenteral nutrition (TPN), 78
Toxic epidermal necrolysis syndrome
        (TENS), 128-137
    causes of, 129-130
    clinical presentation of, 131-132
    defined, 129
    differential diagnosis of, 129, 133-
        134
    epidemiology of, 129
    historical background of, 128-129
    pathophysiology of, 130-131
    pediatric, 163
    prognosis for, 132-133
    treatment of, 134-135
Toxin translocation, 57, 71-72
TPN (total parenteral nutrition), 78
Trace elements, 78
Translocation of toxin, 57, 71-72
TraumaCal on sample admission or-
        ders, 35
Treatment
    admission orders for, 34-39
    by allied health practitioners, 43-44
    central venous pressure catheter
        changes for, 44
    choice of bed in, 44
    debridement and coverage in, 24-
        33, 41
    for extremity burns, 42-43
    for facial burns, 42
    fever workup for, 44
    intravenous antibiotics for, 44
    notes and presentation on, 39-41

Treatment—cont'd
  other issues in, 44
  preoperative evaluation for, 41
  and preparing for discharge to
      home, 45
  for prevention of hypothermia, 24
  psychiatric, 45
  rehabilitation in, 45
  repeat excisions and grafts for, 42
  resuscitation in, 22-23
  step-down burn care in, 44-45
Trunk, escharotomy of, 26
Tube feedings
  for pediatric patients, 166
  on sample admission orders, 35
TwoCal HN, 80

U
Ulcer(s)
  decubitus; *See* Pressure sores
  leg, 123-124
  Marjolin's, 106
Upper airway, damage to, 89
Urinary nitrogen loss, 69-70
Urinary urea nitrogen (UUN), 75
UUN (urinary urea nitrogen), 75

V
Venous access in pediatric patients,
  155
Venous stasis, leg ulcerations from,
  123-124
Ventilation
  airway pressure release, 92
  high-frequency, 91
  for inhalation injury, 91-92
  inverse-rate, 91
  low tidal volume, 92
  management of, 94
  minute, 94, 96
  pressure-control, 91, 92

Ventilator management, 92-94
Ventilator setting and CO_2 level,
  96-97
Ventilator settings
  for pediatric patients, 168-169
  on sample admission orders, 38
Ventilatory equations, 98-100
Vital signs
  pediatric, 159, 165
  on sample admission orders, 34
Vitamin(s), 77
Vitamin C in wound healing, 105
Volume replacement, 22-23
VT (tidal volume), 91

W
Wet-to-dry dressings for mechanical
  cleansing, 118
Whirlpool for mechanical cleansing,
  118
Wound(s)
  common pathogens in, 57-58
  decontamination of, 106
  infected, 54-58, 60-64, 122
  initial management of, 58-60
  with loss of skin, 105-106
  pathophysiology of, 55-57
  preoperative parenteral antibiotics
    for, 61
  systemic antifungal agents for, 64
  tetanus prophylaxis for, 61
  topical antibiotics for, 56, 61-64
Wound care, 54-67
  basics of, 104
  burn patients as unique population
    for, 65
  and chemotherapy, 123
  debridement in, 115
  general (nonburn) inpatient, 103-
    127
  for infected wounds, 60, 122

initial management in, 58-60
for leg ulcerations, 123-124
negative pressure wound therapy
    for, 115-120
for pediatric patients, 161-163
preoperative parenteral antibiotics
    in, 61
for pressure sores, 107-121
products for, 115, 116-120
prognosis for, 121
stages of wound healing and, 104-
    105
surgical coverage in, 121
tetanus prophylaxis in, 61
for tissue damage from radiothera-
    py, 122-123
topical antibiotics in, 56, 61-64
with wound contamination, 106
for wounds with loss of skin, 105-
    106
Wound care products, 115, 116-120

Wound care team, 111
Wound cleansing products, 116-117
Wound closure, 58
Wound contamination, 106
Wound contraction, 106
Wound coverage, 41, 42, 59-60, 121
Wound healing
    chemotherapy and, 123
    with loss of skin, 105-106
    radiotherapy and, 122-123
    stages of, 104-105
. Wound protection products, 119-120
Wound sepsis, 54-58, 60-64

Z
Zinc levels, 78
Zone of coagulation, 7, 8
Zone of hyperemia, 8, 9
Zone of stasis, 8, 9
Zones of burn injury, 7-9

NOTES

NOTES

NOTES

NOTES

NOTES

NOTES

RULE OF NINES

Body diagram for determining total burned surface area (%TBSA)
Numbers (%) are for anterior only and posterior only.

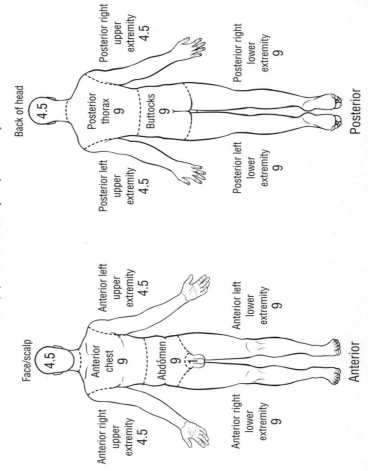